e**X**tensions

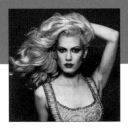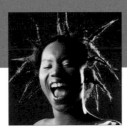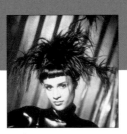

HAIRDRESSING AND BEAUTY INDUSTRY AUTHORITY SERIES

HAIRDRESSING

Mahogany Hairdressing: Steps to Cutting, Colouring and Finishing Hair *Martin Gannon and Richard Thompson*

Mahogany Hairdressing: Advanced Looks *Richard Thompson and Martin Gannon*

Essensuals, Next Generation Toni & Guy: Step by Step

Professional Men's Hairdressing *Guy Kemer and Jacki Wadeson*

The Art of Dressing Long Hair *Guy Kemer and Jacki Wadeson*

Patrick Cameron: Dressing Long Hair *Patrick Cameron and Jacki Wadeson*

Patrick Cameron: Dressing Long Hair Book 2 *Patrick Cameron*

Bridal Hair *Pat Dixon and Jacki Wadeson*

Trevor Sorbie: Visions in Hair *Kris Sorbie and Jacki Wadeson*

The Total Look: The Style Guide for Hair and Make-up Professionals *Ian Mistlin*

Art of Hair Colouring *David Adams and Jacki Wadeson*

Start Hairdressing: The Official Guide to Level 1 *Martin Green and Leo Palladino*

Hairdressing – The Foundations: The Official Guide to Level 2 *Leo Palladino*

Professional Hairdressing: The Official Guide to Level 3 *Martin Green, Lesley Kimber and Leo Palladino*

Men's Hairdressing: Traditional and Modern Barbering *Maurice Lister*

African-Caribbean Hairdressing *Sandra Gittens*

The World of Hair: A Scientific Companion *Dr John Gray*

Salon Management *Martin Green*

BEAUTY THERAPY

Beauty Therapy – The Foundations: The Official Guide to Level 2 *Lorraine Nordmann*

Professional Beauty Therapy: The Official Guide to Level 3 *Lorraine Nordmann, Lorraine Appleyard and Pamela Linforth*

Aromatherapy for the Beauty Therapist *Valerie Ann Worwood*

Indian Head Massage *Muriel Burnham-Airey and Adele O'Keefe*

The Official Guide to Body Massage *Adele O'Keefe*

An Holistic Guide to Anatomy and Physiology *Tina Parsons*

The Encyclopedia of Nails *Jacqui Jefford and Anne Swain*

Nail Artistry *Jacqui Jefford, Sue Marsh and Anne Swain*

The Complete Nail Technician *Marian Newman*

The World of Skin Care: A Scientific Companion *Dr John Gray*

Safety in the Salon *Elaine Almond*

eXtensions

THE OFFICIAL GUIDE TO HAIR EXTENSIONS

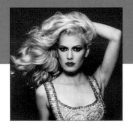 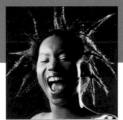 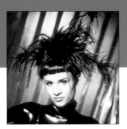

THERESA BULLOCK

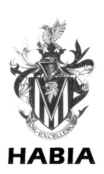

HABIA

THOMSON

Australia • Canada • Mexico • Singapore • Spain • United Kingdom • United States

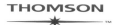

eXtensions: The official guide to hair extensions

Copyright © Thomson Learning 2004

The Thomson logo is a registered trademark used herein under licence.

For more information, contact Thomson Learning, High Holborn House, 50–51 Bedford Row, London WC1R 4LR or visit us on the World Wide Web at http://www.thomsonlearning.co.uk

British Library Cataloguing-in-Publication Data
A catalogue record for this book is available from the British Library

ISBN 1-84480-039-3

Published by Thomson Learning 2004

Typeset by Meridian Colour Repro Ltd, Pangbourne-on-Thames
Printed in Croatia by Zrinski d.d.

Tess

What have you done to me?

I feel young and sexy and full of life!

I was wolf whistled today!

Can't remember the last time that happened!

Every one loves my new hair-do

And they all think you are brilliant!

Thank you

THANK YOU

All my love an all

Mandi

This book is dedicated to Mandi, who wore hair extensions beautifully.

Sadly missed by all who loved her.

contents

foreword

'Your best is not enough – only excellence will do' is just one of the sayings I often use. And nowhere does this ring true but in this excellent and beautiful book by Theresa Bullock. I was astounded by the depth of knowledge Theresa shows throughout the pages and by the images of how wonderful hair extensions look when so expertly crafted.

I remember in the early days, when HABIA was developing the first Level 3 standards, meeting Simon Forbes and Meredith and soliciting their opinions on hair extensions. It was apparent that the potential growth of hair extensions and the different methods of application required a standard. And as HABIA has now delivered national standards for hair extensions, it comes as no surprise to learn that Theresa Bullock came up through the ranks of Dome and Antenna, learning from Simon and Meredith, to become today's hair extensions specialist.

Theresa is not just a hair extension expert, but also an immensely talented trainer and platform artist. Add in the knowledge of salon management, TV appearances, PR skills and her love for research and development and we can see why Theresa is in such demand today.

This is a book that you'll not want to put down and which will feed your desire to go out and learn about hair extensions.

Alan Goldsbro
Chief Executive Officer
HABIA

about the author

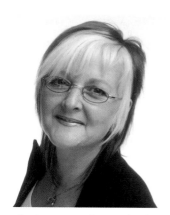

Theresa Bullock has had her own successful hairdressing salon in a high profile, upmarket, high street location. In 1985 she introduced a hair extension service within her own business and was the first extension salon in her area. She continued to teach this service on a freelance basis.

Theresa changed her direction and in 1994 she joined an international hair extension product company. She quickly gained recognition as an international educator and has appeared on television and on platforms around the world, promoting and demonstrating this service at trade fairs, conducting main stage hair shows to large audiences, and has taught distributors, hairdressers and apprentices. Additionally Theresa became a stylist to several celebrities and has travelled worldwide, teaching, promoting and demonstrating hair extensions. Theresa has great enthusiasm for hair extensions, creating outstanding transformations and dream hairstyles for consumers and sharing her knowledge and skills with fellow hair artists.

Theresa is a qualified hairdresser and has committed her whole career to this industry, beginning her training in 1980. She has City & Guilds Ladies' and Gents' Hairdressing – Incorporated Guild of Hairdressers, Wigmakers and Perfumers – Assessors Award D32 and D33 and Master Craftsman in Hairdressing.

Theresa is a member of the Freelance Hair and Beauty Federation (FHBF) and a founder member of the FHBF artistic team, of the Hair and Beauty Industry Authority (HABIA) and the Optime Skills Team as the national and international hair extension expert. She is also a Senior State Registered Hairdresser (SSRH).

Theresa currently is the Principal and Managing Director of aX10 Hair Extension Training. aX10 is an independent training company running courses that teach many extension systems, teaching hairdressers how to create extension hairstyles using real extension hair and synthetic fibre hair.

As the author of this, the first hair extension textbook, Theresa is delighted to have written an aid to all hairdressers who have a desire to learn this exciting and creative service.

acknowledgements

Write, publish and sell the world's first hair extension textbook. What a daunting task! It is all very well coming up with a good idea, but actually fulfilling the task is a very different story. Traditionally, this is the page on which the author thanks everybody who helped achieve the task of completing and publishing this book. However, writing and publishing is just the beginning, as the book must then be sold. Therefore I begin this acknowledgement to you the reader. Thank you for buying this book and I sincerely hope you gain the knowledge you require to be successful with the hair extension service.

TO THE PEOPLE WHO HELPED ME COMPLETE THIS PROJECT

'Behind every good woman is a good man'. In my case that man is Ben, my husband. His encouragement (on my bad days, his nagging) has helped me to reach this goal. Without him I would not have finished on time – timing has never been my strong point, as he will tell you.

Helen Callaway, my sister and also the sales support manager for aX10 Hair Extension Training. A year ago Helen said 'If you don't write this book someone else will' and she has motivated me to get on with it. Helen organises my diary. Thank you for giving me the space to complete this project, and for your constant encouragement and enthusiasm which have kept me focused and on track.

Sharon Forrester, a totally professional lecturer for aX10 – her unconditional faith, support, energy and encouragement have been invaluable.

Jerry King, Andrew Gregory, Joanne Myers, Samantha King and Jackie McShannon are a few of the very skilled hair extension hair stylists I have had the honour of working with. They are wonderful hairdressers and have taught me so much about the extension service. Although I have been a teacher for most of my career, I have been a pupil to these hairdressers. Thank you.

Meredith was my boss at Dome and Antenna; she encouraged me to achieve what most hairdressers can only dream of. Everyone needs a mentor and Meredith was mine. I would not have the knowledge or courage to write this book without her.

Simon Forbes, the man who invented, developed and marketed the first Caucasian hair extension system in 1980. Simon is the founder of this revolutionary service and his creation started me on my path.

Patrick Cameron and Trevor Sorbie. With the publication of their books I saw that hairdressers could also be authors. Both men are an inspiration.

Pat Taylor, my tutor at college. No day passes without my thanking this lovely lady for giving me the foundations of my craft, taking me under her wing and enabling me to believe in myself.

Special thanks to the photographers, make-up artists, models and stylists who helped create the photographic images in this book.

Thank you to the product companies who sponsored pages in this book – without them it would not be published.

The publisher Thomson Learning and HABIA have been a fantastic support.

To the hairdressing industry's trade associations and HABIA for finally recognising that hair extensions are a professional hairdressing service that must have a minimum standard.

The author and publisher would like to thank the following for their contributions to the book:

Anders, Aphrodite (Falkirk), Angela Barnard, Marcello Benfield, Kelly Cooper Barr, Charlie, Cheynes, City & Guilds, Patrick Cameron, Jennifer Cheyne, Jim Crone, Dome (www.domecosmetics.com), Martin Evening, Sharon Forrester, Janet Francis, Great Lengths, Hair and Beauty Industry Authority (HABIA), Hair Direct, HMSO, Michelle Joslin, Suzie Kennett, Ashley Kerr, J.J King, Karen Lockyer, Kathryn Longmuir at Ishoka (Aberdeen), Jackie McShannon, Jack Melville, Heather Miller, Irvine Miskell-Reid, Joanne Myers, Optime, George Paterson, Peter and Bernard (Bathgate), Rainbow Room International Artistic Team (Glasgow), Stuart Phillips Creative Team, Malcolm Willison.

sponsors

aX10 Hair Extension Training

Contact: Theresa Bullock
aX10 PO Box 568
Richmond
Surrey
TW9 2GX
Tel/Fax: 020 8274 8290
Email: ax10head@blueyonder.co.uk
www.theresabullock.com

BaByliss Pro

The Conair Group Ltd
Prospect Court
3, Waterfront Business Park
Fleet
Hampshire GU51 3TW
Tel: 08705 133 192
Fax: 01252 813028
Email: fay_cowell@conair.com
www.babyliss.co.uk

American Dream

Unit 5, Acton Vale Industrial Park
Cowley Road, Acton
London W3 7QE
Freephone: 0800 085 2294
Tel: 020 8740 1383 or 020 7743 0206
Fax: 020 8740 0966
Email: jas@sahneys.com
www.ad-hairsolutions.com

Cinderella Hair

Unit A
The Sunbeam Centre
Sunbeam Road
Park Royal
London NW10 6JP
Tel: 020 8965 3777
Fax: 020 8965 6333
Email: enquiry@latrend.com
www.savagelily.com

BALMAIN
PARIS

Euro Hair Fashion UK Ltd

PO Box 144
Hailsham
BN27 3YT
Freephone 0800 781 0936
Tel 01323 842288
Fax 01323 449211
Email: info@eurohair.co.uk
www.eurohair.co.uk

(HD) HAIR DEVELPMENT (UK) Ltd.

Hair Development (UK) Ltd

247 Mile End Road
London E1 4BJ
Tel: 020 7790 3996 or 020 7790 4567
Fax: 020 7790 3621
Email: hair@hair-development.com
www.hair-development.com

Mane Connection: Hair Extension & Enhancement System

Little Bourton House
Southam Road
Banbury
OX16 1SR
Tel: 01295 757 410
Fax: 01295 757 401
E-mail: sales@maneconnection.co.uk
www.maneconnection.co.uk

RACOON
no1 in hair extensions

Racoon International

PO Box 1458
Southam
Warwickshire CV47 0WS
Tel: 01295 770 999
Fax: 01295 770 199
Email: e@racooninternational.com
www.racooninternational.com

WELLA

Wella UK

Wella Road
Basingstoke
Hampshire
RG22 4AF
Tel: 01256 320 202
Fax: 01256 471 518
Email: info@wella.co.uk
www.wella.co.uk

introduction

This book, as far as I know, is the first hair extension textbook to be written. It is the theory text or underpinning knowledge supporting *Unit H23 – Provide hair extension services (option group 1)* found in the National Vocational Qualification (NVQ) Level 3 hairdressing. It is written as the definitive guide for students studying NVQ Level 3 and for any hairdresser who wants to offer the hair extension service to clients. The unit covers the hair extension skills required to reach a minimum standard in order to provide the service to clients.

This book covers the main outcomes expected in Unit H23.

The hair extension service is as comprehensive a subject as modern day colouring perming and relaxing, requiring equal amounts of training and education. It is a skill that can not be learnt from a video, book or manual alone, but a combination of all three training skills will enable a practitioner to begin offering this service to clients.

My aim in writing this book is to impart years of knowledge and skill to the hairdressing profession, to unravel the mysteries surrounding the completion of extension hairstyles and to introduce this exciting service to the hairdressing industry with which I have been involved all my working life.

The hair extension service is here to stay and is now recognised as a professional hairdressing service, along with this, the first textbook.

chapter 1

THE HAIR EXTENSION SERVICE

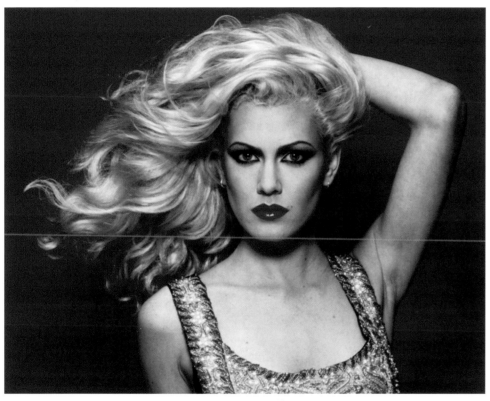

Hair by J. J. King, photography Michelle Joslin

Learning objectives

- understand the hair extension service
- introduce the four hair extension systems available in the marketplace
- the pros and cons of the differing hair extension systems
- show that the hair extension service achieves four separate hairstyles
- study the quantity of extension hair and the minimum length of natural hair required for each extension hairstyle

The **hair extension** service attaches **synthetic fibre extension hair** (fibre)
or **real human extension hair** (real hair) into a client's natural hairstyle
using a variety of application methods. Hair extensions are **strands of
extension hair** approximately the size of a highlight or **wefts** or **strips** of
extension hair that are prepared specifically to be attached onto natural hair.

The **hair extension service** can be used to create a variety of hairstyles.
It is as comprehensive a service as modern day colouring and perming and
is considered the third technical hairdressing service, requiring the same
amount of time for technical training.

Technical training covering theory, knowledge and practical skills is
required. This service is very adaptable and can be used to create colour
effects, body, volume, length and very radical hairstyles like braids and
dreadlocks.

There are four main **hair extension systems** used to apply strands or wefts
of extension hair into a client's hairstyle:

1 Hot-bond
2 Cold-fusion
3 Braiding
4 Sewing

HOW THE HAIR EXTENSION SYSTEMS WORK

Hot-bond extension system

Also called the hot system, this is the most commercial and most widely
used extension system in the UK. It relies on heated tools that melt **polymer
resins** or synthetic fibres creating hard **bonds** which attach extensions at the
root area of the natural hair. The hot system is most suitable for use on
Caucasian, **Asian** or **Oriental** hair types because it enables an extension
practitioner to apply individual strands of extension hair, thus allowing the
finished hairstyle to be free-flowing. This gives it an authentic natural look.
This system is easy for the practitioner to cut and style and for the client to
brush and style the extension hairstyle at home.

The hot system can be used on **African-Caribbean hair**, although there are
other systems that are better suited.

The tools required

The hot system uses three specific tools: the first is a **hot-bond extension
dispenser** (dispenser). This works by depositing a hot polymer resin
adhesive at the root end of the fibre or real extension hair; both resin and
extension hair can be attached to natural hair, creating a hard bond.

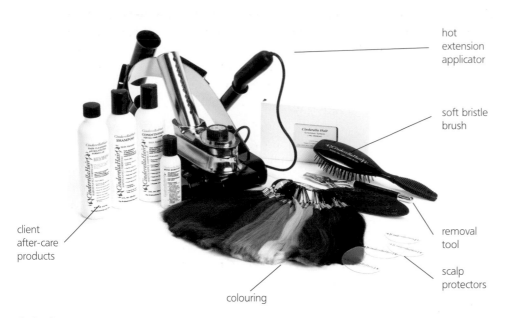

hot extension applicator

soft bristle brush

removal tool

scalp protectors

colouring

client after-care products

Cinderella

The second is a **hot extension applicator** (applicator). This tool is suitable to heat a fibre or real extension hair strand – both of which have polymer resin adhesives already deposited on the end of the extension strand. These are called **pre-bonded** extension strands. The applicator is designed to heat the pre-bonded extension and melt the polymer resin in order to secure the extension to the natural hair at the root area; this creates a hard bond.

The third tool used in the hot system is a **heat clamp** which is used to heat fibre; it melts the fibre that is applied to the natural hair. The melted fibre forms a hard bond at the root area of the extension and natural hair to secure the extension in place.

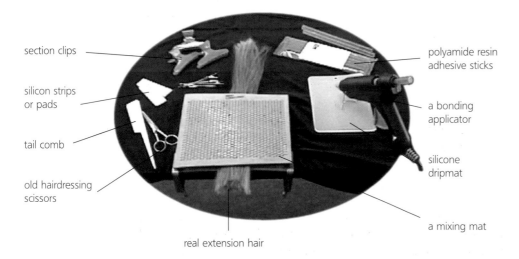

section clips

silicon strips or pads

tail comb

old hairdressing scissors

polyamide resin adhesive sticks

a bonding applicator

silicone dripmat

a mixing mat

real extension hair

Mane Connection Enhancement System

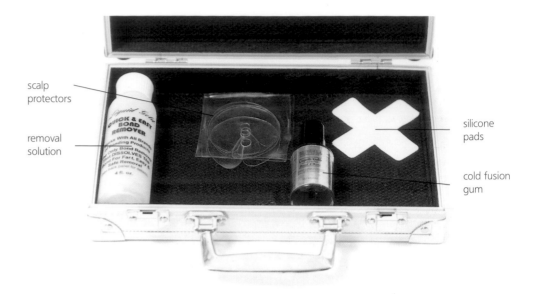

scalp protectors

removal solution

silicone pads

cold fusion gum

Hair Development (UK) Ltd

Cold-fusion extension system

This system relies on **cold adhesives** or **cold solutions** to hold the strands or wefts of extension hair in place on natural hair. Cold-fusion solutions are **spirit**, **latex** or **rubber-based gums**, or **toupee tapes**. These products are adhesives and they fuse together to hold the fibre or real extension hair on to natural hair. Cold systems can create bonds and can be used on all hair types.

Cold fusion is widely used in African-Caribbean extension applications. It is becoming a popular choice for Caucasian, Asian and Oriental hair types, as the system becomes more sophisticated and product research and development continues.

Plaiting or braiding extension systems

This is a method of braiding fibre or real extension hair into a natural hairstyle. There are several different types of braid that can be made by a practitioner to attach the extension hair and we will show examples of this later in this book. This extension system gives a very strong hairstyle image that is highly decorative. The braiding system can be used on all hair types but is most suitable on African-Caribbean hair types and *thick* Caucasian, Asian and Oriental hair types.

Sewing extension systems

This is a system where wefts of fibre or real extension hair are sewn onto **scalp plaits** called **cornrows** or **cornbraids** using a **curved needle and thread**. The braiding and sewing extension systems originated from African-Caribbean hairdressing and have been used by this ethnic group for hundreds of years. Sewing systems are best suited on African-Caribbean hair types; however, as with the braiding system, it can cross over into thick and curly Caucasian, Asian and Oriental hair types.

CHOOSING A HAIR EXTENSION SYSTEM

In order to choose which extension system or systems to work with, it is useful to know the advantages and disadvantages of each system and to take them into consideration before introducing it as a service.

The **hot-bond extension system** allows a practitioner to create large or small extension strands, depending on the thickness or fineness of natural hair. The hot systems stay looking good in natural hair for up to three months.

HEALTH AND SAFETY

Follow the manufacturer's instructions for use and maintenance
Water boils at 100°C, and the hot bond tools range in temperature between 120°C–220°C – they are exceptionally hot. The tools and resins will cause serious burns to the practitioner or client if misused. Always read and follow the manufacturer's instructions for use and maintenance of these tools.

The hot system allows the extensions to be put in individually so that the hairstyles are free-flowing and look very authentic. This system enables a practitioner to mix a variety of extension hair colours together to match a natural hair colour exactly.

The hot-bond extension system is suitable for all hair types and is easy to remove.

The heated tools range in temperature, heating up to between 120°C–220°C, which means that they get exceptionally hot and will burn the practitioner and the client if misused.

The **removal** of the hot systems can take a long time – from one to three hours for a whole head. Some bonds can leave tiny knots in the natural hair at the root area and these can be difficult to comb out.

On African-Caribbean hair, removal of the hot-bond extension system can be difficult, as this hair type is delicate; breakage during removal is a strong possibility. Always take test strands before using the hot system.

Cold-fusion systems do not require heat, thus eliminating the risk of burns. These systems are exceptionally quick to apply – a lengthened hairstyle can take only 45 minutes to one hour to complete. Practitioners can mix the extension hair colours to match the client's natural hair colour exactly. Cold-fusion systems can be used on all hair types. This system is used to add wefts or create bonds for free-flowing extension strands. Some of the cold-fusion products are also very fast to remove, taking only 15–20 minutes. Cold systems adhere to natural hair for one to three months depending on the cold product used. Cold-fusion tapes are perfect for fine thin delicate hair types.

Unfortunately some cold-fusion products can be very sticky and messy to use and therefore difficult to work with efficiently. Clients can also prove very allergic to these products. Although severe allergies are rare they are a fact of life, and these products can cause **anaphylactic shock**. When planning to use the cold system do **skin sensitivity tests** on *every client*.

Removing the cold systems on fine Caucasian hair and African-Caribbean hair can be very difficult because the gum will fuse to the hair and penetrate into the hair shaft. Conduct strand tests to check natural hair strength during removal before continuing with a cold system. Tapes will hold in place for four to six weeks and clients will need to visit the practitioner regularly when wearing tapes. This particular technique is recommended for fine thin hair as it does not fuse to the natural hair.

HEALTH AND SAFETY

Skin sensitivity test
Before conducting a skin sensitivity test ask clients whether they suffer from allergies: this will give a clear indication of whether to go ahead with the sensitivity test. If practitioners are in doubt do not continue with the procedure.

The test
Clean an area behind a client's ear, dab a small amount of the cold fusion product just behind the ear and leave this product for 24 hours. Check the skin in this area for a rash or abnormal sensitivity. If the test proves sensitivity is present do not go ahead with the use of the product.

HEALTH AND SAFETY

Traction alopecia
Constant tight braids will cause **traction alopecia** – hair loss around the hairline due to continual pulling and strain on the hair shaft of natural hair. Do not braid hair tightly at the hairline, ensure a braided hairstyle is *not* worn continually and give natural hair time to grow before repeating a braided extension hairstyle.

The **braiding extension system** gives a very strong decorative look to a hairstyle. Most of the braiding systems are best suited for African-Caribbean hair textures. Braids can be placed through the natural hair or just one or two can be used to add into hairstyles as decoration – e.g. for a bridal hairstyle. Braiding systems last for three months and must then be removed.

The disadvantage of braiding is that Caucasian, Asian and Oriental hair textures tend to be straight and have flat **cuticle layers** enabling **fibre braids** to slide down the hair shaft. Braids can look scruffy on these hair types.

Braids are attached using tight **scalp tension** that can cause **tension spots**, discomfort and breakage. For this reason it is important to test strand before a full application, checking for **scalp sensitivity** and natural hair strength.

The drawback to the braiding system is the time – a whole head of braids can take anywhere from 6 to 22 hours to apply.

The removal of the braiding system is also similarly time-consuming, as the practitioner must unravel every braid individually.

The **sewing extension system** is a very quick application and the removal is very quick and easy. This is a perfect application for African-Caribbean hair customers who completely change hairstyles and image frequently. Wefts are most commonly used on African-Caribbean hair and look good in thick curly Caucasian, Asian and Oriental natural hair.

The practitioner needs to be very skilled at scalp plaits to use the sewing system as the end hairstyle can be quite bulky at the roots. This system is best suited for African-Caribbean hair types as the bulk at the root area is easily disguised. Although it can be used on Caucasian, Asian and Oriental hair, its use is recommended for temporary extension hairstyles, e.g. for a bride or for photographic and session work.

Sewing systems can put strain on natural hair and are quite heavy, causing breakage or alopecia on fine delicate hair. Curly and thick hair can withstand this strain easily. Strand test the natural hair to check it can take the strain.

Sewing systems last for four to six weeks: as braids loosen and lift away from the scalp the wefts become visible; additionally, the stitches can become loose and unravel. Salon visits must be frequent when using the sewing system.

Before introducing an extension system to a hairdressing business research the clientele. Investigate what percentage of your business will be Caucasian, Asian, Oriental or African-Caribbean. There is a divide between the four systems: the hot-bond and cold-fusion systems are best suited for Caucasian, Asian and Oriental hair and the braiding and sewing systems are best suited for African-Caribbean hair types. Understanding the four extension systems will help potential extension practitioners to decide which will be the best system or systems for their business.

HAIR EXTENSION HAIRSTYLES

Hairdressers can create many varied hairstyles for their clients using the hair extension service. The hair extension hairstyles fall into four categories:

1 Hair additions
2 Hair enhancements
3 Hair extensions
4 Hair alternatives

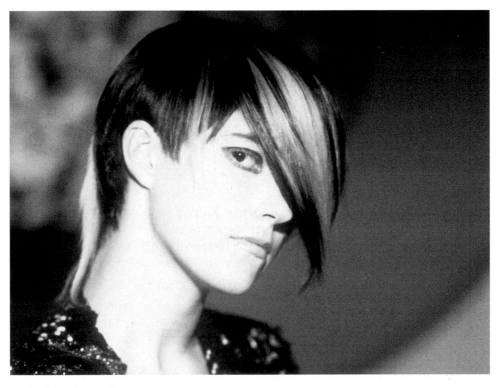

Hair by Ashley Kerr at Cheynes

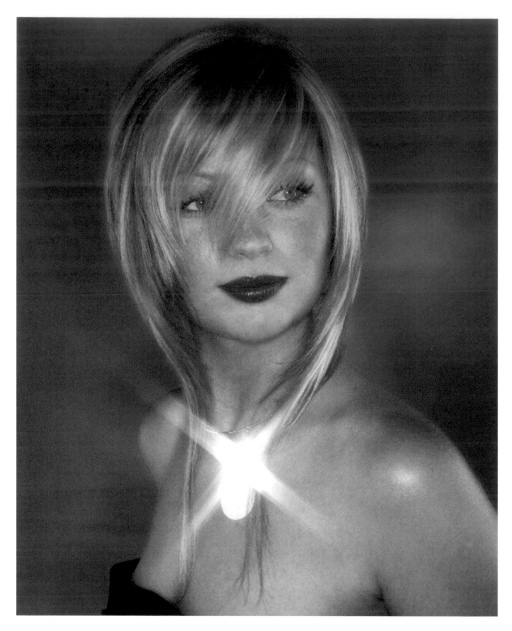

Optime

A **hair addition hairstyle** is created using one to fifty individual extension strands. One extension strand weighs approximately 1 gram, so to achieve a hair addition hairstyle 1–50 grams of fibre or real extension hair on a weft will be needed. The addition service consists of extension strands attached into a client's natural hairstyle to create highlights, lowlights, and flashes of colour, decorations and adornments. Hair additions can be used to colour hair when a client is anxious about using a chemical colouring process – additions are used to add **neon colours** that glow in the dark under ultra-violet light or **fantasy colours** that cannot be achieved with a chemical process. Additions give 'Colour without commitment'. Additions are used in bridal hairstyles and long, hair-up, hairstyles as adornments. Natural hair needs to be the minimum of 7.5 cm (3 inches) long to apply additions.

A **hair enhancement hairstyle** is created from 50–150 strands of fibre or real extension hair loose or on a weft. Hair enhancements thicken natural hair to give body or improve the look of a natural hairstyle. Enhancements are ideal for a client who has fine hair to add thickness. They are also suitable for clients who have little time to style or dress their hair, as the enhancements will help to hold a client's hairstyle in shape for longer. Enhancements are the fastest growing and most sought after service using extension hair, as clients require subtle authentic, undetectable results. Enhancement hairstyles give body; natural hair needs to be 12.5 cm (5 inches) long to apply enhancements.

A hair extension hairstyle is created using extension hair that is the same colour as a client's own hair. Use from 150–250 individual strands of fibre or real extension hair to give client a lengthened hairstyle and from 150–250 grams of extension hair that is on a weft to create an extended hairstyle. The lengthened hairstyle is the most commonly asked for hairstyle with this service. Natural hair needs to be a minimum of 15 cm (6 inches) long to create extension hairstyles.

A **hair alternative** hairstyle is **textured fibre** or real extension hair that is made by the practitioner into a **braid**, a **dreadlock** or any design that cannot be created by nature with natural hair. Alternatives completely cover natural hairstyles. Hair alternatives are viewed as quite extreme radical changes to a client's image. Use 100–250 strands of fibre or real extension hair, use between 100–400 grams of extension hair. Alternatives fulfil

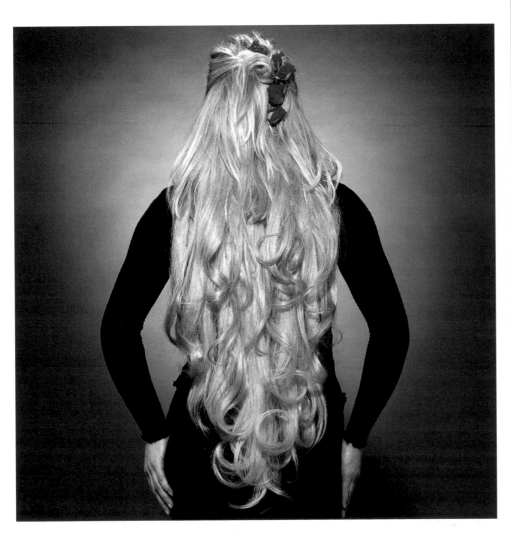

Patrick Cameron

FASCINATING FACT

Famous hair alternative hairstyle
Boy George sported one of the most famous hair alternative hairstyles, wearing an early dreadlock and braided multi-textured hairstyle when he hit the UK number one spot with his hit single Karma Chameleon. His hairstyle was created at Antenna Hair Salon in Kensington, London, the Mecca for hair extension hairstyles at that time. Antenna's proprietor, Simon Forbes, invented the world's first hair extension application, in 1980, for Caucasian hair – Monofibre™ hair extensions using a heat clamp. Boy George wore the first dreadlocked hairstyle ever seen on a public stage on Caucasian hair; his image was at that time cutting edge, ground-breaking and breathtakingly radical. These looks are commonplace today thanks to Simon Forbes.

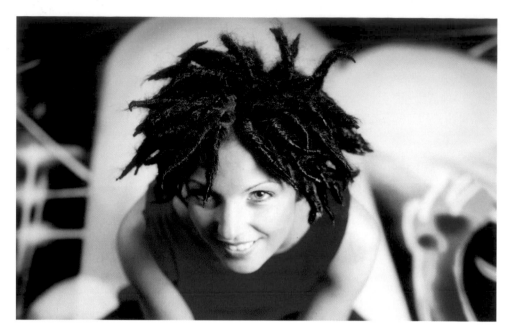

Hair by Jackie McShannon, photography Charlie

hairstyle fantasies, defying nature. Natural hair needs to be a minimum of 7.5 cm (3 inches) long to create alternative hairstyles.

This chapter has given an overview and foundation of the hair extension service, covering its uses and differing systems. We have explained that there are a number of extension applications and four hairstyle categories that this service can be used to create.

Knowledge review

1 Which hair extension system is currently the most commercial in the UK marketplace and why?

2 What are cold-fusion adhesives made of?

3 Which extension systems are recommended to be applied on African-Caribbean hair and why?

4 When would you conduct a skin sensitivity test?

5 For how long should a hair extension hairstyle be worn by a client?

6 Describe a hair addition hairstyle.

7 Describe a hair alternative hairstyle.

8 How many extension strands do you need to create a hair enhancement hairstyle?

9 How many grams of extension hair will you need to create a hair extension hairstyle?

10 Who else can you name (apart from Boy George) who wears or has worn a hair alternative hairstyle?

11 Who, in 1980, invented the world's first Caucasian hair extension system?

chapter 2

PREPARING FOR THE HAIR EXTENSION SERVICE

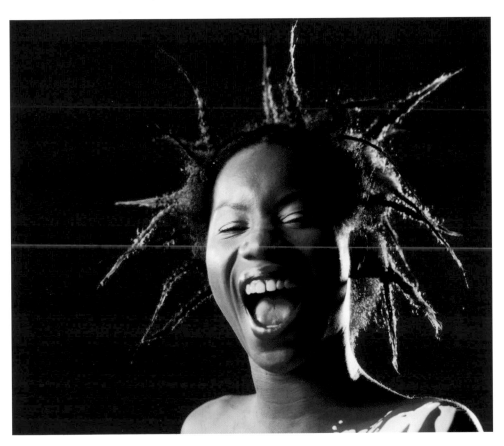

Hair by Joanne Myers, photography Michelle Joslin

Learning objectives

- the legal requirements to put in place before offering a hair extension service
- aspects of the insurance cover needed when offering this service
- how to source and access professional hair extension training from recognised accredited training bodies

Learning objectives continued

- the training qualifications available for this service
- understand that practical and theory training is required and that this takes the same period of time as colour or perming education
- learn the safe working practices necessary to perform this service
- potential risks and hazards involved
- health and safety legislation in place for hairdressing and the specific acts that relate directly to the hair extension service

INSURANCE AND LEGAL REQUIREMENTS

Contact an insurance company before introducing the hair extension service. Some insurers do not automatically cover the hair extension service; it comes under the same category as chemical treatments such as colouring and perming. Insurance companies are strict with their coverage of the service. Over the last two decades, there have been enormous insurance claims for hair loss, breakage to natural hair, alopecia, infection, burns and allergies. An insurance company will ask for evidence of professional training in this field of hairdressing before effecting **insurance cover**.

The law requires a hairdresser to use reasonable care and skill in carrying out their business. If a client is injured, the hairdresser will be **liable for negligence**. Comprehensive insurance coverage is a legal requirement to all practitioners offering hairdressing services, including hair extensions.

The law makes an employer liable for the wrongful acts of the employee, provided that the wrongful act was committed in the course of the employee's employment. Hairdressers should confirm with their insurers that they and their employees are covered by insurance. If a hairdresser is negligent the insurance company will pay the ensuing claim on behalf of the employer but is empowered in some circumstances to take steps to recover their loss from the employees themselves.

A hairdressing business has a liability towards any person who is injured by the equipment they use if the injury was due to a **defect in the equipment** of which they knew or ought to have known. As with all hairdressing equipment, it is important to keep the products and tools used in this service well maintained and to repair or replace the tools if they are faulty. If the tools used were faulty and an injury occurs, the practitioner would be solely responsible.

These are the insurance and **legal requirements** to look into before introducing the hair extension service into a business. Contact the National Hairdressing Federation (NHF), Freelance Hair and Beauty Federation (FHBF) or the Hairdressing and Beauty Industry Authority (HABIA), who are linked with reputable insurance companies that specialise in insuring hairdressers and beauty therapists.

REMEMBER !
If a client is injured the hairdresser will be liable for negligence. Negligence is proved when a practitioner has not followed legal safe and professional working standards.

REMEMBER !
Obtain **Public and Employers liability** insurance to cover all hairdressing services.

REMEMBER !
Insurance companies will not cover you for badly maintained equipment!

PROFESSIONAL TRAINING AVAILABLE FOR THE HAIR EXTENSION SERVICE

Insurance claims against those providing hair extension services are generally due to lack of professional training that meets minimum standards or failure by a practitioner to follow a manufacturer's recommendation. Insurance companies may ask to see evidence of a qualification or a certificate of participation before giving cover. Various types of training are available for the hair extension service.

Courses can be taken at a **Further Education College**. The hair extension education is an optional unit, Unit H23, found in NVQ Level 3. Additionally an Advanced Hair Extension Certificate Specialist's Award can be gained from City and Guilds. Contact HABIA for a list of colleges offering these qualifications.

Private hair extension training companies are accredited or working towards accreditation by the Hairdressing and Beauty Industry Authority (HABIA) to

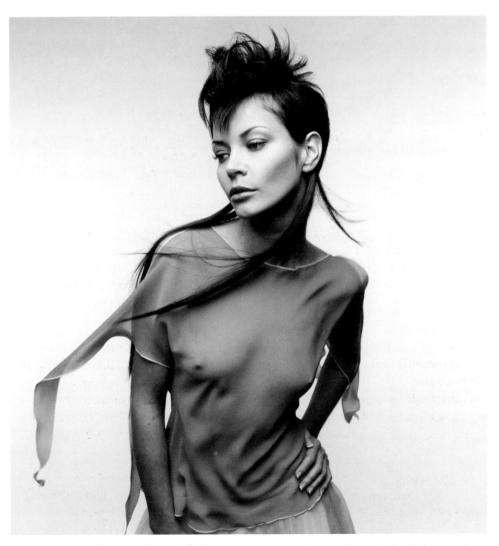

Hair by Rainbow Room International Artistic Team, Glasgow, make-up Janet Francis, clothes styling Angela Barnard, photography Martin Evening

ensure they reach minimum standards of training. These **private extension-training companies** are independent, teaching a variety of hair extension techniques, applications and procedures. They are not allied to one particular extension system or product company but specialise in this field of hairdressing. Look for HABIA approved courses or Continued Personal Development (CPD) accreditation when seeking private training. Accredited certificates are attained after attending these courses, ensuring that each delegate has reached a minimum standard. Contact HABIA for the list of private CPD-accredited hair extension training companies.

Training can be found via product companies that manufacture and supply the tools, products and equipment for specific hair extension systems. Certificates of participation are attained from the product companies giving evidence that a delegate has attended training for this specific extension system following all manufacturer's recommendations and standards set out by the product companies organising this training. Find these product companies listed or advertising in the hairdressing trade press and hairdressing literature.

Product company training videos are available. Watching a training video and reading a manual will only be an aid to practical training and certificates are generally not issued with this form of learning. There is no substitute for **practical training**, which will enable a practitioner to perform the extension service safely and to a minimum standard.

There are many courses, seminars, workshops and demonstrations available to teach the different hair extension systems. Attend as many varied courses as possible, as this ensures the practitioner can choose exactly the right extension system before introducing this service to a business.

Professional training for the hair extension service is as comprehensive in theory and in practical work as colouring and perming and any other technical service that practitioners offer in the hairdressing business. It therefore requires exactly the same amount of training.

On completion of hair extension training delegates should be able to:

- provide a consultation service for hair extensions
- apply hair extensions by heat sealing – both real and synthetic extension hair
- apply extensions by cold fusing – both real and synthetic extension hair
- apply hair extensions by sewing real and synthetic hair
- apply extensions using braiding methods
- cut and style extensions to suit temporary and permanent methods of attachment
- recommend and provide relevant client aftercare products to clients
- complete the safe removal of hair extensions without causing damage to client's natural hair
- work effectively and safely whilst adding hair extensions
- plan and prepare hair extension hairstyles
- use a variety of cutting and styling tools using several cutting and styling techniques to finish the hair extension hairstyles.

TOP TIP ✔

Videos alone are not considered professional courses – always gain practical and theory education alongside videos.

With any hair extension training, whether with an independent training company, via a product company or through the further education route, delegates should cover the theory of hair extensions. Use this textbook to cover the theory and use the worksheets covering client consultations and client aftercare.

The theory must cover the **contra-indications of hair extensions**, Natural hair analysis, safe working practices, planning and placement, **extension sizes**, cutting and styling, consultation aftercare and maintenance aspects of the hair extension service.

> **REMEMBER** !
>
> Seek recognised education from professional training establishments who cover the theory and practical aspects of this service.

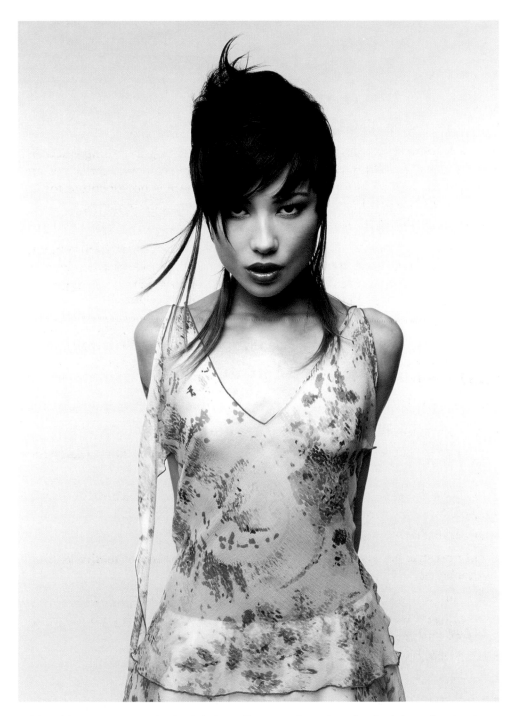

Hair by Rainbow Room International Artistic Team, Glasgow, make-up Janet Francis, clothes styling Angela Barnard, photography Martin Evening

POSSIBLE RISKS WHEN USING THE HAIR EXTENSION SERVICE

As with all hairdressing services there are possible risks, but the hair extension service has unique areas that are potentially hazardous to **health and safety**. Understanding these risks will enable a business to complete a comprehensive risk assessment ensuring that all legal legislation is covered. When taking the hair extensions service into your business, write a **health and safety policy**. When employing five or more staff on the premises this policy becomes a requirement by law. Managers and employers have a responsibility and requirement to address or demonstrate that they can identify potential hazards in the hair extension service. They must work towards eliminating them so that it is not a hazard to the general public and staff, or minimise the risk to the public and staff by taking precautionary action. Managers and employers must be able to evaluate the processes and activities that occur at work, record the result and define the precautionary action to be taken. There are very helpful booklets available on this subject that can be accessed from hairdressing trade associations.

This general health and safety policy should include details of the storage of chemicals, checks of all electrical equipment by a registered qualified electrician, fire escape routes and evacuation procedures. On this policy name the person responsible for health and safety in the salon, as well as the person responsible for first aid. Everyone in the salon should know the location of the **first aid kit** and the **accident book**. A copy of this policy should be given to each employee who should read it and ensure that they understand it.

The hot-bond extension systems

The tools used with this system reach very high temperatures, and can cause serious burns when used incorrectly or accidentally touched. The heated tools have a temperature range from 120°C–250°C. When applying this system ensure gowns are used to protect clients from accidental spillage of the hot polymer resins dispensed from these tools. Use **scalp protectors** or **scalp shields** when bringing hot tools to the client's head (see page 38).

Do not bring the hot applicators that dispense heated resins directly to the client's head.

Ensure that the heated extension tools such as dispensers, applicators and heat clamps are placed on a flat stable work surface while performing the extension service.

Ensure all electrical heated applicator cables and wires are safely removed from walkways and are not on the floor or around the practitioner or client's feet. These tools must be placed out of reach of clients and untrained staff or guests. Ensure the correct polymer resin adhesives are used in the correct applicator tools.

TOP TIP

Always follow the manufacturer's product recommendations for using these tools.

The cold-fusion extension system

Cold-fusion systems may cause allergic reactions. Conduct a skin sensitivity test and strand test before applying this system on a client (see page 6).

(see page 6).

> **TOP TIP**
>
> Always follow manufacturer's instructions when using cold-fusion products.

> **REMEMBER** !
>
> When applying this system ensure gowns are used to protect clients from accidental spillage.
>
> Work in well-ventilated areas as some of the cold-fusion products omit strong chemical fumes and in some cases the products are **flammable**.

The braiding extension system

The braiding extension system can cause an injury called tension spots. These occur on a client's scalp if the braids are plaited too tightly. Tension spots are created when the hair is pulled excessively at the scalp area, putting a strain on the hair bulb. Tension spots easily become **infected**, as the **skin pores** are opened by the excessive **tension**, and **bacteria** regenerates in this environment. It can cause the client severe discomfort and medical treatment may be required. Traction alopecia, the loss of hair due to tension applied to the hair, is a risk with this system.

> **TOP TIP**
>
> Keep comprehensive client record cards and consultation sheets for further reference.

The sewing extension system

When working with the sewing system, sharp needles are used and could inadvertently pierce a client's skin. Care must be taken with this system to ensure that a curved needle is always used to reduce the risk of injury. Sewing with thread can put excessive tension on the scalp area causing tension spots. Traction alopecia is a risk with this system.

General risks associated with the hair extension service

- Keep nails trimmed, hands clean and hand jewellery to a minimum because of the risk of passing on infections with dirty hands and nails.
- Nails and jewellery can easily get caught in the extension hair, which is uncomfortable and painful. If jewellery gets caught in the extension hair it can result in having to cut it out.
- There is a risk of **cross-infection** when reusing extension hair.
- When applying hair extensions, clothes must be comfortable and not too tight because you can be standing for a long time.
- Always wear comfortable shoes that will enable you to stand virtually stationary for 5–10 hours.

> **HEALTH AND SAFETY**
>
> Never take extension hair out of one client and place that extension hair onto a different client.

- Consider the practitioner's posture and the position of a client when working with extensions, ensure that you are working on either a **gaslift chair** or a **hydraulic chair** so that you can move your client up and down. This will lessen the chances of suffering **repetitive strain injury** to your back and neck.

- The environment you work in when performing the hair extension service must be immaculately clean. Workstations, hairdressing trolleys, any work surfaces and the surrounding floor area must be kept spotless.

- Extension hair is very slippery if left on the floor and you could inadvertently slide on it, even though you are not moving around very much. For this reason, extension hair must be constantly swept up.

- When applying the hair extension service on a client ensure that proper gowns or capes are worn so that the client is protected from hair clippings, accidental spillage of hot polymer resins, cold-fusion products or removal solutions. All of these products can cause burns or allergic reactions.

- Extension hair that has fallen on the floor must not be applied into a client's natural hair.

- Always ensure tools are sterilised and cleaned when they have been in contact with a client before using them on another client.

> **REMEMBER** !
>
> Always read and follow the manufacturer's instructions for use of all tools, equipment and products involved in the hair extension service.

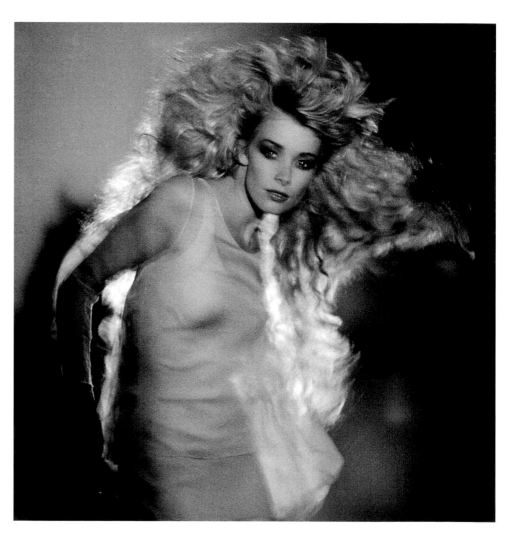

Hair by Jennifer Cheyne

- The use of razors or razor blades is common with the hair extension service. Ensure disposal of these is in a container designated for this purpose.

> **TOP TIP**
>
> A 'sharps' box must be used to dispose of razor blades. It must have a screw top lid and when full it must be disposed of properly.

- Ensure that your place of work or study is well-ventilated while using extension **removal solutions** as these products can be highly flammable or omit an odour that in a non-ventilated area can become nauseous.
- Ensure there is no smoking or naked flames while using removal solutions and cold-fusion spirit gum products as these are flammable.
- Always clear up any spilled chemicals immediately.
- If using a product that needs special care and attention when handling ensure that you wear protective equipment, for example **latex** or **rubber gloves**.

> **FASCINATING FACT**
>
> Extension removal products can remove nail extensions, nail polish, wood varnish and can melt holes in plastic trolleys and plastic plumbing pipes.

> **TOP TIP**
>
> Test the extension chemicals on protective gloves before usage, as some of these products will melt holes in the gloves therefore rendering the protection useless.

> **REMEMBER**
>
> Wear rubber or latex gloves when handling chemicals to reduce the risk of allergy, **dermatitis** or infection.

If you are not working on a client performing the hair extension service, it is still important that you stay alert and ensure that you keep your work environment safe. Often accidents are avoided by others spotting potential hazards.

HEALTH AND SAFETY REQUIREMENTS

Legislation is provided within the Health and Safety at Work Act 1974:

> All employers and employees are required to take reasonable care for their personal health and safety and of any other people who may be affected by his or her actions or omissions and to cooperate with their employer so that their employer can fulfil an obligation by compliance to the current UK and EC health and safety requirements.

Ensure that your salon or workplace displays the Health and Safety at Work Act 1974. This act covers several health and safety regulations that affect hairdressers and their work.

Refer to Chapter 1 of *Professional Hairdressing – the Official Guide to Level 3*, fourth edition by Martin Green and Leo Palladino (published by Thomson Learning) for a comprehensive explanation of this Act.

Have a basic understanding of first aid. Ensure that your business has a first aid kit available and antiseptic cleanser, eye bath, eye-cleansing lotion, cotton wool, burn ointment, disposable bags and disposable gloves. It is vitally important to have these items in your first aid kit.

HEALTH AND SAFETY FOR HAIRDRESSERS

COSHH RISK ASSESSMENT

HABIA

Staff Member Responsible:		Date:		Review Dates:	
Hazard	What is the risk?	Who is at risk?	Degree of risk High/Med/Low	Action to be taken to reduce/control risk	
Aerosols (list aerosols used in your salon)	These can contain flammable gases and irritant chemicals. There is a risk of fire, explosion and intoxication.	Everyone in the salon, but in particular the user of the aerosol and the client.	Low	Look for aerosols with non-flammable gases if possible. Do not expose to temperatures above 50 C. Do not pierce or burn containers. Do not inhale.	
Nail polish remover (list products used in your salon)	Irritant to the skin and eyes. Moderately toxic if swallowed or inhaled.	Beauty therapists, juniors, trainees and clients.	Medium	Store in a cool place. Reseal after use. Do not use on damaged or sensitive skin. Avoid breathing in. Never place in an unlabelled container.	

EXAMPLE

HSIP 2a

All accidents and emergency aid given must be documented in an accident book. A qualified first aider or a medical practitioner must treat serious accidents.

When working with the hair extension service it is especially important that you are aware of the control of substances hazardous to health or COSHH regulations 1999.

You don't need to know this legislation by heart, but you will need to know its basic contents. Hairdressing employers are required by law to make

HEALTH AND SAFETY FOR HAIRDRESSERS

COSHH ACTION PLAN

HABIA

Staff Member Responsible:		Date:			Review Dates:	
Problem requiring attention	Priority High/Med/Low	Action to be taken	Staff Member Responsible	Completion Date Target	Completion Date Actual	Result
Staff complaining that Xedos Acid Perm is making clients and staff feel nauseous and faint.	HIGH	Contact manufacturer for advice. Look for alternative product. Do not use this product.	Mary Murphy	30/11/98	22/11/98	Manufacturer can only suggest using product in well ventilated area. Product will not be used in salon again. Newline Acid Perm has been ordered and the manufactuer has not experienced
						any bad reactions with this. Staff to be trained to monitor its use carefully and report any problems to Mary Murphy.

EXAMPLE

HSIP 2c

assessments of the exposure to chemical substances used in the salon that are potentially hazardous to health.

The purpose of a **COSHH** assessment in the salon is to ensure the working environment is as safe as possible. A hazardous substance is a product that can cause harm to a body.

Make sure that you have these substances clearly marked and labelled for staff who have been trained to work with the chemicals and products and, more importantly for untrained staff, to avoid confusion which could result in a serious accident.

> **REMEMBER** !
>
> Produce a COSHH assessment focusing on hair extension products and chemicals.

HSE
Health & Safety Executive

Health and Safety at Work etc Act 1974 [?]
The Reporting of Injuries, Diseases and Dangerous Occurrences Regulations 1995

Click here for report guidance

Report of an injury or dangerous occurrence

Filling in this form
This form must be filled in by an employer or other responsible person.

Part A

About you

1 What is your full name?

2 What is your job title?

3 What is your telephone number?

About your organisation
4 What is the name of your organisation?

5 What is its address and postcode?

6 What type of work does the organisation do?

Part B

About the incident
1 On what date did the incident happen?

2 At what time did the incident happen?
(Please use the 24-hour clock eg 0600)

3 Did the incident happen at the above address?

Yes ☐ Go to question 4

No ☐ Where did the incident happen?
☐ elsewhere in your organisation – give the name, address and postcode
☐ at someone else's premises – give the name, address and postcode
☐ in a public place – give details of where it happened

If you do not know the postcode, what is the name of the local authority?

4 In which department, or where on the premises, did the incident happen?

F2508 (05.00)

Part C

About the injured person
If you are reporting a dangerous occurrence, go to Part F. If more than one person was injured in the same incident, please attach the details asked for in Part C and Part D for each injured person.

1 What is their full name?

2 What is their home address and postcode?

3 What is their home phone number?

4 How old are they?

5 Are they
☐ male?
☐ female?

6 What is their job title?

7 Was the injured person (tick only one box)
☐ one of your employees?
☐ on a training scheme? Give details:

☐ on work experience?
☐ employed by someone else? Give details of the employer:

☐ self-employed and at work?
☐ a member of the public?

Part D

About the injury
1 What was the injury? (eg fracture, laceration)

2 What part of the body was injured?

Next Page

Also please make special note of the **Electricity at Work Regulations** 1989. This regulation covers the installation and maintenance of electrical equipment and tools in the workplace. On an annual basis all electrical equipment must be inspected, tested and recorded to show that it is in safe working order.

This book will be highlighting health and safety procedures in the use of the hair extension service you will see these in HEALTH AND SAFETY boxes. What we have covered here are the general health and safety and safe working practices required to perform the hair extension service within a business based on the tools, products, chemicals and equipment that are used.

SUMMARY

Before undertaking the hair extension service in a hairdressing business ensure that:

- Full comprehensive insurance covers the legal aspects of the business.
- You take practical and theory training for this service – there is no substitute for practical training to enable you to perform it safely. Gain training from training bodies who reach recognised industry minimum standards. All of the training points mentioned will be covered in detail throughout the course of this book.
- You conform to the health and safety regulations that are in place under the law.

These issues must be addressed *before* undertaking the hair extension service in a hairdressing business.

Knowledge review

1 How does a client prove negligence against a practitioner?
2 What qualifications can be achieved covering the hair extension service?
3 Where do you gain professional hair extension education?
4 What does CPD accreditation mean?
5 List three approved hairdressing trade associations.
6 Where do you find the theory information required for this service?
7 List five headings that should be covered during hair extension training.
8 Give two examples of potential risks whilst performing hair extensions. Give two examples of potential hazards whilst performing hair extensions.
9 What is the Health and Safety at Work Act?
10 What does COSHH mean? Make a COSHH assessment list for your workplace.

chapter 3

TOOLS AND PRODUCTS

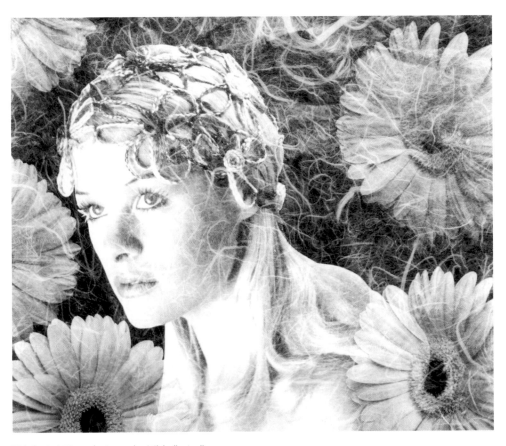

Hair by J. J. King, photography Michelle Joslin

Learning objectives

- introduction to the unique vocabulary of the hair extension service
- understand the use of each tool and product
- the importance of a checklist of equipment for each hair extension system
- client aftercare products required for this service

HAIR EXTENSION PRODUCTS AND TOOLS

Synthetic fibre extension hair

This is a man-made fibre that has been specifically designed as the hair to use to create hair extension hairstyles. It is an **acrylic** fibre that is heat sensitive.

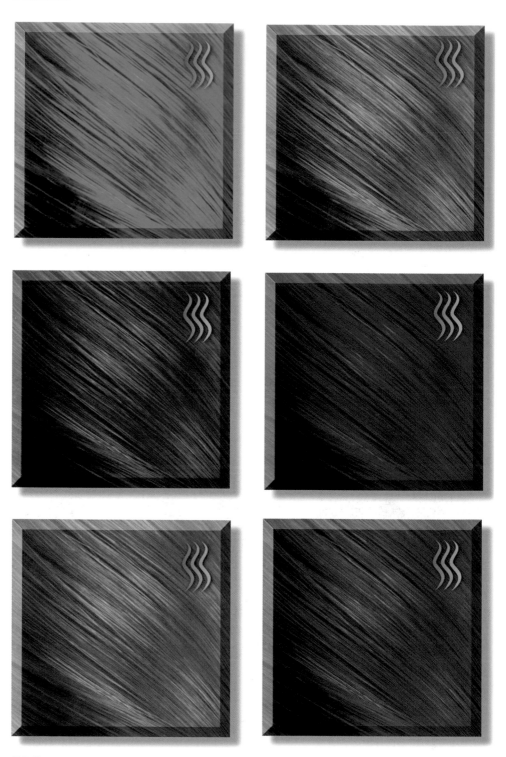

Hair Direct

The fibre is manufactured in a range of natural colours, from black to lightest blonde and a range of tonal colours: gold, copper, red and burgundy. Fibre is manufactured in a range of fantasy colours: red, green, blue, yellow, orange, violet and purple together with an assortment of neon colours that glow under ultraviolet light. Synthetic fibre is also manufactured in a range of pre-blended colours. This means that the natural and tonal colours or the fantasy colours are mixed together, giving a huge range in the colour spectrum to choose from.

Fibre is packaged in 30 gram–100 gram packets, and 1 kilo boxes. Fibre hair comes in varied lengths, starting at 35 inches/87 cm to 60 inches/150 cm. Fibre is manufactured in many **structures**.

To create natural hairstyles the structures are called:

- straight hair, soft wave, deep wave, curly, spiral or ringlets

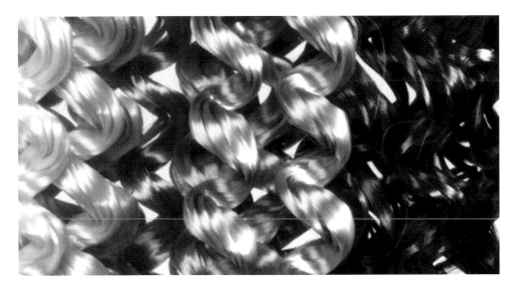

Spiral curls American Dream

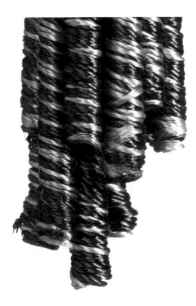

Ringlets American Dream

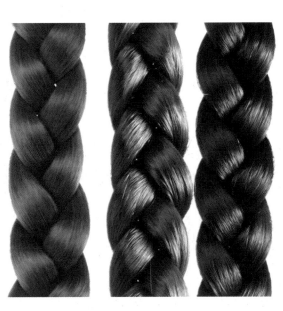

Pre-made fibre braids American Dream

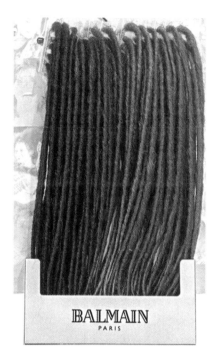

Pre-made fibre dreadlocks
Pierre Balmain, courtesy of Euro Hair
Fashion, world licensed manufacturer of
Balmain Hair Extensions

To create alternative hairstyles the structures are called:

● Pre-braided and pre-made **dreadlocks**, **crimped** or **crinkled hair**, structured at the factory. Fibre used for braiding is called **jumbo fibre**; it is frizzy in texture and grips natural hair, ensuring that the braid does not slide down the hair shaft.

To create African-Caribbean hair styles the structures are called:

● Afro curl and relaxed African-Caribbean textures.

Some fibres are coated with a cuticle layer. This layer is designed to strengthen the fibre and improve the quality; it makes fibre looks less plastic and shiny. Fibre hair can be bought at a range of prices – the more processes the fibres go through, the more costly it is to manufacture. The high quality coated fibres are more expensive than fibre that has no cuticle layer.

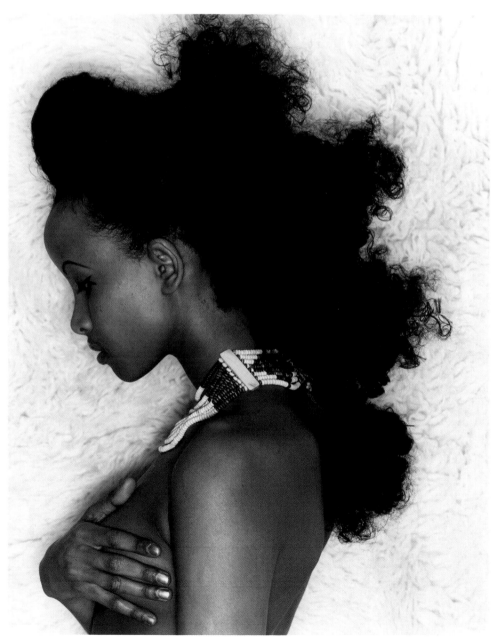

Hair by George Paterson, photography by Malcolm Willison, make-up by Suzie Kennett, products by Wella

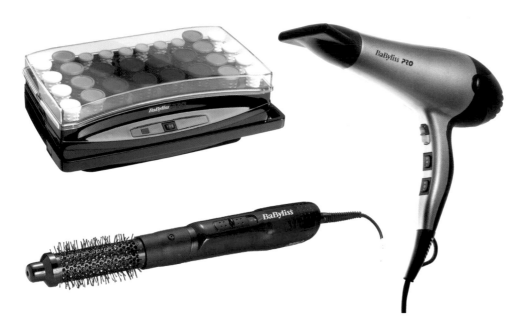

Heated rollers, airstyler and hairdryer   BaByliss

Fibre is a synthetic man-made acrylic and is affected by heat. The use of heated electrical hairdressing tools will damage the fibre. All electrical hairdressing styling tools must be used on a medium heat setting when blow drying, setting or styling. The use of heated rollers is suitable for fibre extensions.

TOP TIP

Fibre hair is used to create hair alternative hairstyles, as these are unnatural hairstyles. Use fibre to create the different styles when real hair will not be able to give the results required.

FASCINATING FACT

Many of the hair extension product companies are working towards perfecting a heat-resistant fibre. This fibre will look, feel and behave like real hair. Once they have solved the heat sensitivity problem, hairdressers will be able to buy fibre that will be almost identical to real hair.

Fibre is prepared in what is called **bulk hair**. Bulk hair is loose hair with a band tied at either end to contain the fibre, preventing tangling before application. Fibre is also prepared on a **weft**. This is a strip of hair that looks like a curtain or sheet of hair. Fibre wefts are machine sewn.

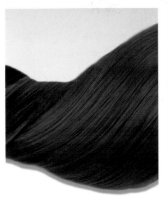

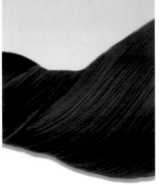

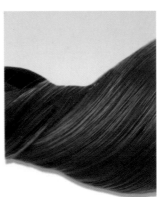

Hair Direct   Hair Direct   Hair Direct

Real extension hair

Real hair is Asian, Oriental or European hair collected from India, China and Eastern bloc European countries. It is collected as fallen or brushed, gathered together, and then sold to hair factories to be prepared for use in wigs, toupees and hair extensions. Real hair is also donated or sold to religious temples and then sold on to hair factories or is sometimes sold directly to hair factories from independent people.

Once the real hair has arrived at the hair factories it is cleansed in a mild **caustic soda** solution to remove any infestation that may be present. After cleansing the hair is lightened then permed if a soft wave or deep wave structure is required. The hair is then tinted to match the colour rings that are produced to match the required extension hair colours.

During the cleansing, tinting and perming process the real hair must be kept root point correct. Root point correct means placing the real hair with the root end and tip end together. Real hair must not be prepared upside down, as this will lead to matting of the real hair. The cuticle layers will lock together and become impossible to pull apart!

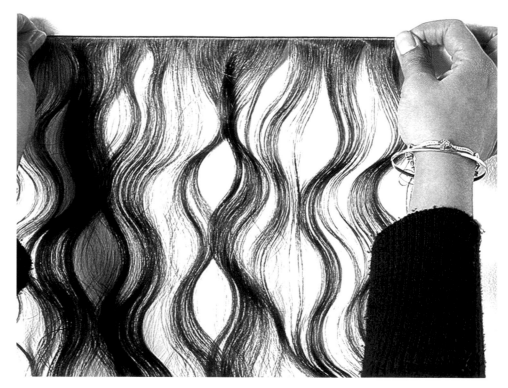

Real hair, machine sewn into a weft. This hair has been coloured and permed into a soft wave structure   American Dream

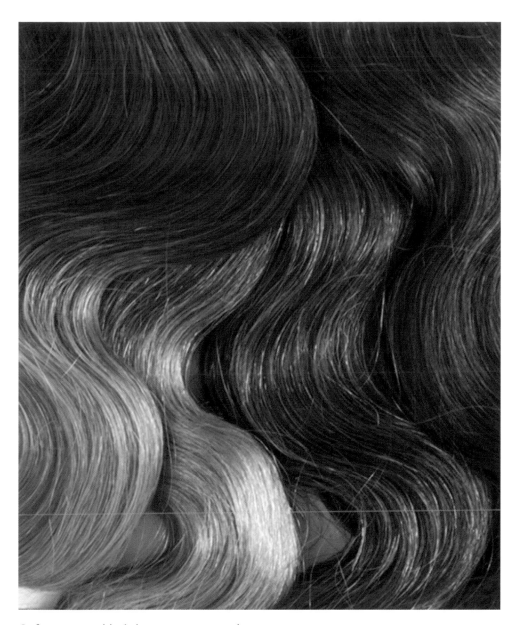

Soft wave real hair in a two-tone colour   American Dream

Real hair is available as **virgin hair**, this means it has not been chemically treated. Real virgin hair is generally only available as European hair types.

Real hair comes in a range of **virgin natural colours**, **tinted natural colours**, **tinted tonal colours**, **tinted fantasy colours** and also **two-tone colours**, for example, black at the roots and blue at the tips.

Unless working with virgin hair, real hair has to be cared for as chemically treated hair. Real hair is packaged in 1–4 ounce packets (approximately 25–100 grams) and comes in varied lengths from 10 inches (25 cm) to 24 inches (60 cm).

Real hair is produced in many structures:

- **Silky straight**, **soft wave**, **deep wave**, **curly**, **spiral curl** and **ringlet curl**.

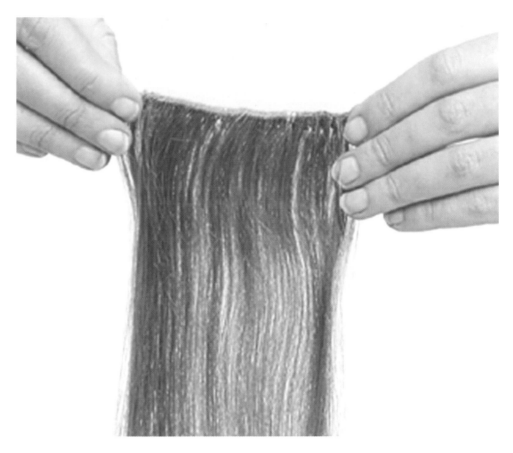

A hand-sewn weft of real hair   Pierre Balmain, courtesy of Euro Hair Fashion, world licensed manufacturer of Balmain Hair Extensions

- You can get real hair structures that are the same as straightened African-Caribbean hair.

Real hair can be prepared on a weft. This is a strip of natural hair that looks like a curtain or sheet of hair. Wefts are sewn into a weft of hair; it can be machine or hand-sewn.

Hand-sewn wefts are considered superior as they experience little or no **shedding**. Wefts are sewn at the root area, which holds the hair on a strip.

Real hair is also prepared in what is called bulk hair. Bulk real hair is loose hair with a band tied around the root area of the hair. The hair is tied and packed cuticle correct.

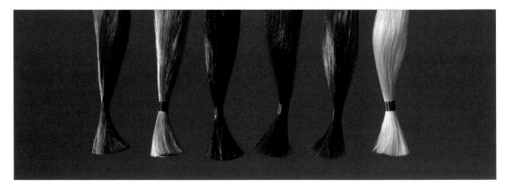

Real extension hair tied in bulk   Racoon

European hair is more expensive than Asian or Oriental hair, purely because it is more difficult get hold of. The price depends on length and shade: the longer it is and the lighter the hair colour, the more expensive it will be. This is because the lighter the hair, the more processes it has gone through and more manpower has gone in to producing it. Virgin European hair is the most expensive hair on the market because of its rarity.

Pre-bonded extension hair

These are strands of fibre hair or real hair, packaged in individual pieces of 10–25 extensions. These individual strands are pre-bonded, which means they have a polymer resin adhesive on the root end. The adhesives are attached during the processing and manufacture of the extension pieces.

Pre-bonded strands come in a variety of structures: straight, wavy, curly, braided, dreadlocked, and crimped in 60 cm (35 inch) lengths.

Pre-bonded **diamond crystal** strands are also available as a hairstyle decoration.

TOP TIP

There is a vast amount of hair in the marketplace. Contact extension product companies, and obtain brochures or look at their websites to see what is available before selecting the correct product for your requirement.

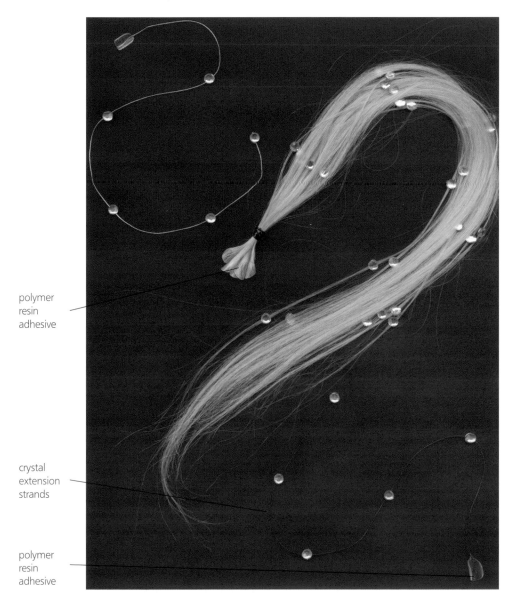

polymer resin adhesive

crystal extension strands

polymer resin adhesive

Pre-bonded real hair and crystal extension strands   Cinderella

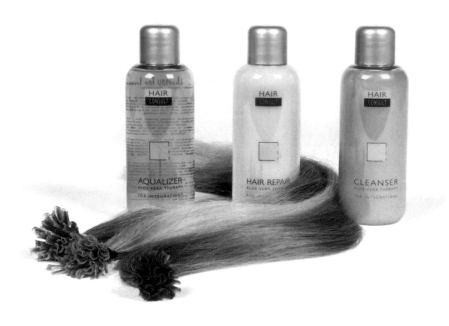

Client aftercare products and pre-bonded extension strands   Pierre Balmain, courtesy of Euro Hair Fashion, world licensed manufacturer of Balmain Hair Extensions

Colour rings or colour shade charts

Colour rings are small swatches of real or fibre hair colours. Colour rings are necessary when working with the hair extension service. They help when ordering extension hair for a client and by placing them up against the client's natural hair colour they are used to select the hair colour required for your client.

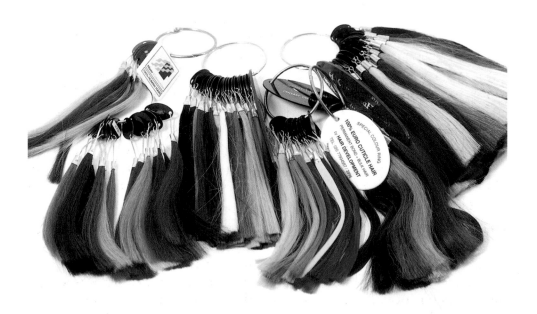

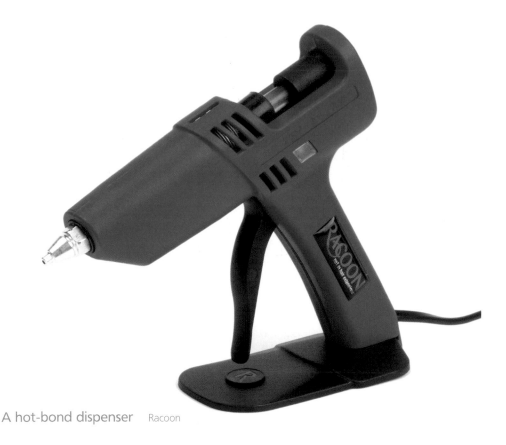

A hot-bond dispenser   Racoon

PRODUCTS, TOOLS AND EQUIPMENT REQUIRED FOR THE HOT-BOND EXTENSION SYSTEM

The hot-bond extension system has three heated tools to choose from in order to apply extensions.

- The hot-bond extension dispenser (dispenser) deposits a hot **polymer** resin adhesive onto the end of either fibre or real extension hair. The polymer resin is put into the tool and dispenses at 180°C.

- The hot extension applicator (applicator) is suitable to heat pre-bonded fibre or real extension hair. These strands have a polymer resin adhesive deposited on the end of the extension. Applicator temperatures range between 80°C–140°C.

- Heat clamps have two hot tips. The temperature ranges from 140°C–220°C. This heat has to be quite specific At the correct temperature it will heat fibre, melting it together to create a hard bond at the root area of the extension.

When purchasing heated tools, read the manufacturer's instructions for use. These instructions will, amongst other very important issues, explain how to clean them properly. It is recommended that the heated tools are to be packed away in a case or airtight container when not in use. This ensures that they are kept safe, out of the reach of untrained hands and this reduces any risk of damage. If heated tools are damaged repair or replace them immediately.

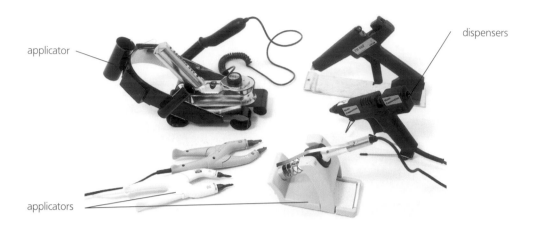

applicator

dispensers

applicators

Polymer resin adhesive sticks or cartridges (sticks)

Polymer resin adhesive sticks are packaged in airtight packets of 5–10 sticks.

Spirit gum or anti-slipping agents

Used when working with a heat clamp. This product is only suitable to use when melting fibre. Fibre hair slips down the hair shaft, and **spirit gum** or **anti-slipping agent** will prevent this from happening so it is important to use them when working with fibre. These are **water-soluble** products similar to those used to attach false beards and moustaches in film and theatre.

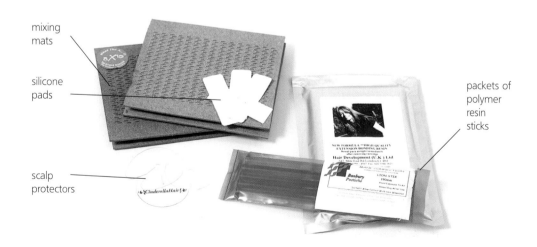

mixing mats

silicone pads

scalp protectors

packets of polymer resin sticks

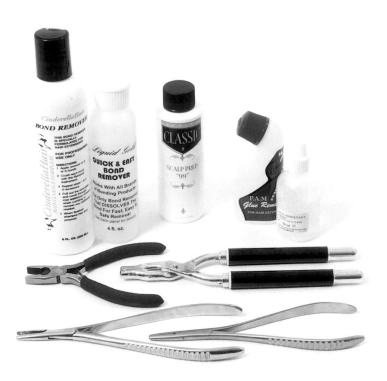

Bottles of removal solutions and removal tools

Removal solutions

Differing product companies recommend different removal solutions. Later in the book we will show you removal techniques and methods to work with some of the removal solutions. Removal solutions are made of **acetone**, **oil** or **alcohol**.

Removal tools

The removal tool is a small pair of pliers. The pliers are designed to crush the adhesive bonds that keep the extensions in place. Removal tools are supplied in starter kits and there are a variety of designs available.

There are client aftercare products for use with the hot-bond hair extension system including a selection of suitable products to care for the adhesive bonds that hold the extensions in place.

Incorrect aftercare products can break bonds down very quickly by dissolving them. Suitable client aftercare products should be recommended to prevent the bonds from dissolving or slipping out of the client's hair during shampooing and conditioning.

PRODUCTS, TOOLS AND EQUIPMENT REQUIRED FOR THE COLD-FUSION EXTENSION SYSTEM

The cold-fusion system does not require heated tools. As the name implies, this system uses cold adhesive products that attach fibre or real extension hair to a natural hairstyle.

Cold-fusion solutions are spirit, rubber or latex-based gums or **bonding tapes**. They have a variety of names. See Chapter 8, Kaori – hair additions and Mia – hair extensions, for demonstrations of their application.

When working with the cold-fusion extension system, *specific removal solutions are needed*. Both cold-fusion products that attach the extension hair and the removal solutions are patented to the companies that manufacture them. It is imperative that only the removal solution that is recommended for a specific cold-fusion adhesive is used. The removal solutions are acetone, alcohol or oil-based. These solutions break down the cold-fusion adhesives to enable the extensions to slide out.

Clients need specific aftercare products that are suitable to care for the cold-fusion adhesives. These aftercare products prevent the adhesive dissolving. Clients must use correct aftercare products for the duration of the cold-fusion extension hairstyle.

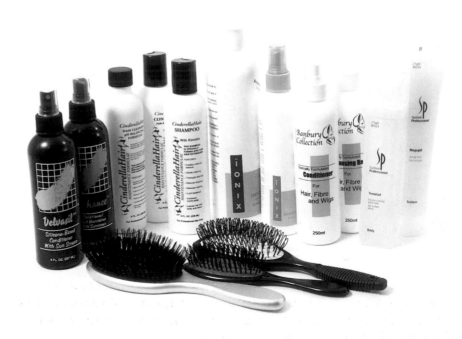

Client aftercare products and soft bristle brushes

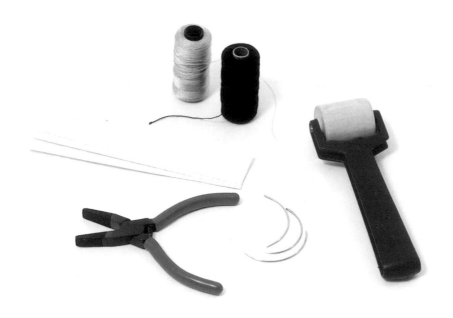

Tools, thread, toupee tape, and curved needles

PRODUCTS, TOOLS AND EQUIPMENT REQUIRED FOR THE BRAIDING EXTENSION SYSTEM

Synthetic fibre hair is the most suitable hair for this system. It is cheaper and will stay in the client's natural hair. You will need a needle and **thread**, **rose wire**, cold-fusion adhesives or a heat clamp.

Heat clamps are used to seal the end of the braid preventing the braided extension from unravelling. Client aftercare products suitable to care for the braided extensions are required for shampooing and conditioning natural and extension hair.

FASCINATING FACT

Rose wire is a very fine wire that can be bought from florists. It is used to tie off the end of braids and assists with threading beads onto braids.

PRODUCTS, TOOLS AND EQUIPMENT REQUIRED FOR THE SEWING EXTENSION SYSTEM

Fibre or real extension hair prepared on a weft or in bulk, suitable to be sewn or stitched into the client's natural hairstyle; a curved sewing needle and a thread that is suitable to be used to stitch natural hair and extension hair together will be needed for sewing systems.

As with the three other systems, specific client aftercare products suitable to care for the extension hair used to create the desired hairstyle and the client's natural hair will be required.

TOP TIP

Thread can be purchased from the appropriate hair extension product companies.

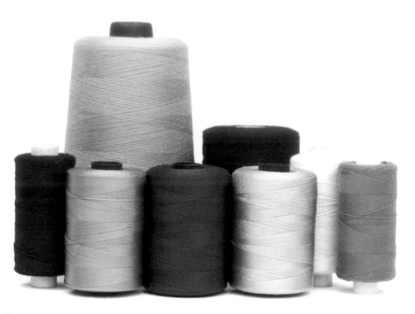

American Dream

OTHER TOOLS AND EQUIPMENT REQUIRED

Silicone pads

Small, heat-resistant finger protectors. Silicone is a product that is heat-resistant and these pads are small sheets of silicone approximately 2 cm wide and 6 cm long.

Silicone pads are designed to wrap around hot adhesive and to roll a polymer resin bond to the same size as a grain of rice. The polymer resin is dispensed onto the root end of extension hair. It is then taken to a small piece of the client's natural hair; using the silicone pad wrap it around the adhesive and roll the adhesive into a bond. This attaches the extension to the client's hair. See Chapter 8 for silicone pad usage.

Silicone pads are used with the hot-bond extension system and the cold-fusion extension system. Cold-fusion adhesives are very sticky but the silicone rolls the bond and the sticky products do not adhere to it.

Protective scalp shields

These are plastic discs approximately 5 cm in diameter with a small hole in the centre designed to draw out the client's natural hair. Protective scalp shields are used when applying extension pieces into a client's natural hairstyle. The shield protects a client's scalp when using hot tools close to the scalp. Scalp shields protect the client from the hot polymer resin drips and hot pre-bonded extensions. It is also used to keep client's natural hair sections clean and to prevent any travelling hairs getting caught in the adhesive bonds of the hair extensions. In Chapter 8 we will be using protective scalp shields during the application of the extension systems.

HEALTH AND SAFETY
Polymer resin adhesive is dispensed from a bonding dispenser at 180°C. Contact with skin will result in a third degree burn.

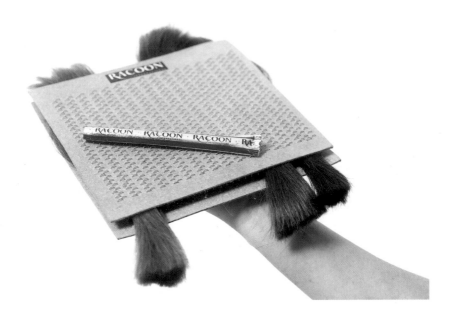

Bulk real hair, polymer resin stick and mixing mat

Mixing mat

A 12 cm by 12 cm flat mat with small metal teeth pierced through it. Use two mats with one placed on top of the other so that the teeth interlock. The mixing mat is for holding real extension hair, cuticle correct, in place while applying the extensions.

Place two or three different colours of real extension hair onto the mixing mat, put the second mixing mat with the teeth interlocking on top and draw the natural extension hair out of it. This will help to mix two extension hair colours together.

CLIENT AFTERCARE PRODUCTS REQUIRED FOR THE HAIR EXTENSION SERVICE

It is important to recommend the correct client aftercare products for use with the different hair extension systems. Some shampoos and conditioners can break adhesives down, allowing the extensions to slip out causing the hair extension hairstyle to fail. Therefore client aftercare recommendations are absolutely vital. Most of the product companies manufacture and supply a range of aftercare products with their system.

Clarifying shampoo

Clients must shampoo their hair with a **clarifying shampoo**. This is a deep-cleansing shampoo. It removes oil, **sebum**, styling products, wax or deposits left on a client's natural hair. It must be used prior to applying hair extensions and continue to be used for the duration of the hair extension hairstyle. This shampoo should be used with every extension system.

Reconstructive conditioner

A rinse-out **reconstructive conditioner** should be used on real extension hair (Asian, Oriental or European hair). A reconstructive conditioner is a conditioner that works inside the structure of the hair shaft. It is important that a reconstructive conditioner is used on real hair because this hair has been chemically treated before it is used in a hair extension hairstyle and its structure is in a weak state and is **porous**. These conditioners are designed to work on the inside of the hair shaft to strengthen it and should be applied to a client's extension hair once or twice a week. The reconstructive conditioner will care for a client's own natural hair, keeping it strong to enable it to hold the extensions in place as well as strengthening the extension hair.

The reconstructive conditioner must be applied to the mid-lengths and ends of the client's natural hair and extension hair. Avoid applying it to the **bonded root area** or where the hot-bond or cold-fusion adhesives sit as these conditioners can soften the bonds.

De-tangling spray

De-tangling spray is recommended when a client is wearing fibre hair. When used daily and sprayed lightly on the synthetic fibre hair it will reduce any static electricity. It is important to reduce static electricity as it produces heat that can damage the surface layer of the fibre extension hair. It also functions as a de-tangler for fibre hair, as the name suggests. Those product companies who specialise in fibre manufacture supply this spray.

Equalising/pH-balanced solution

Equalising/pH-balanced solution is a liquid product that is **pH-balanced**. This means that it has the same pH value as hair and skin.

The solution is designed to close the cuticle layers of Asian, Oriental or European real hair. This is important because chemical treatments on human extension hair damage and open the natural cuticle layer. If the cuticle layers remain open the natural hair can mat together. Equalising solutions help to keep the surface of the real hair flat, therefore reducing tangling and matting. The real hair becomes smooth, making it easier to style and dress.

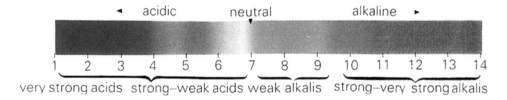

Leave-in conditioner

Leave-in conditioner is designed to moisturise and condition natural hair as well as real extension hair. It is very easy to use and generally quite light. Avoid applying the leave-in conditioner onto the adhesives or the bonded root area where the adhesives have been applied.

Soft bristle brush

To be used with all extension systems and hairstyles. It is designed to thoroughly brush through natural and extension hair, taking with it any loose hairs. If loose hairs are left at the root area of extension hairstyles they will entwine, causing tangling and matting. Brush extension hairstyles with a **soft bristle brush** at least once a day.

STYLIST'S EQUIPMENT CHECKLIST FOR THE HAIR EXTENSION SERVICE

- cutting comb, pintail or **tail comb**
- hairdryer or airstyler and heated rollers
- straighteners, crimpers and heated electrical tools for real hair
- flat section clips
- old pair of hairdressing scissors to cut the extension hair; thinning scissors – razor and razor blades
- a soft bristle brush and a selection of round brushes or blow-drying brushes
- a flat stable work surface
- an area to display client aftercare products.

All of the tools and products explained and listed in this chapter can be purchased from hair extension product companies and local hairdressing suppliers. Product companies sell starter kits for the extension systems and most of the tools and equipment needed are included in the kits.

> **TOP TIP**
>
> Do not use a good pair of hairdressing scissors on extension hair, as extension hair will blunt them.

TOOLS AND PRODUCTS REQUIRED FOR EACH EXTENSION SYSTEM

Equipment	Hot-bond extension systems	Cold-fusion extension systems	Braiding extension systems	Sewing extension systems
Real extension hair	*	*		*
Fibre extension hair	*	*	*	*
Pre-bonded extensions	*			
Hot dispenser	*			
Hot applicator	*			
Heat clamp	*			
Spirit gum or bonding tape		*		
Rose wire			*	

Red stars (*) represent the tools or products for this system

Equipment	Hot-bond extension systems	Cold-fusion extension systems	Braiding extension systems	Sewing extension systems
Curved needle & thread				*
Polymer resin adhesive sticks	*			
Silicone pads	*	*		
Soft bristle brush	*	*	*	*
Removal tool	*			
Removal solutions, cottonwool, rubber gloves	*	*	*	*
Mixing mat	*	*		*
Cutting comb, pintail or tail comb	*	*	*	*
Hairdryer or air styler	*	*	*	*
Flat sectioning clips	*	*	*	*
Hairdressing scissors, thinning scissors	*	*	*	*
Razor and razor blades	*	*	*	*
Protective scalp shields	*	*		
A colour ring or colour shade chart	*	*	*	*
Selection of round brushes or blow drying brushes	*	*	*	*
Flat stable work surface	*	*		
Hairdressing trolley	*	*	*	*
Client aftercare products	*	*	*	*

Red stars (*) represent the tools or products for this system

Knowledge review

1 What is extension fibre made of?

2 What is a weft?

3 What is bulk hair?

4 Where does real extension hair come from?

5 What are the chemical processes undertaken before real hair is ready to be used as extension hair?

6 What is a pre-bonded extension?

7 What is a colour ring?

8 Name the three heated tools that are used in the hot-bond extension system.

9 What is removal solution?

10 What client aftercare products are required for:
  • Fibre hair?
  • Real hair?

chapter 4

HAIR EXTENSION APPOINTMENT TIMES

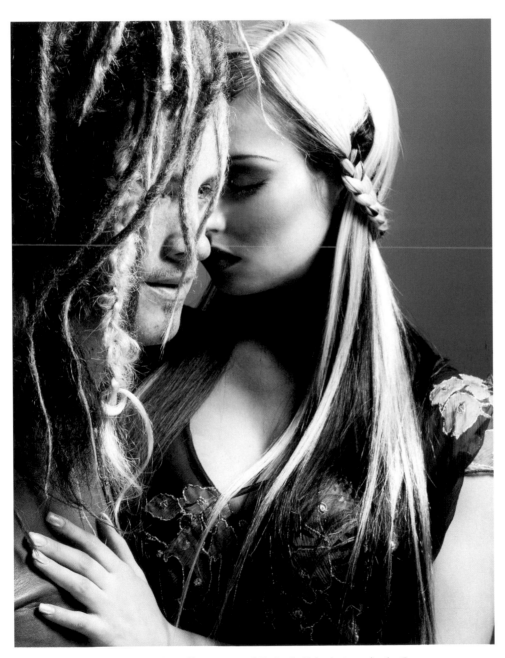

Hair by Sharon Forrester and Heather Miller courtesy of Cinderella Hair, photography Jim Crone

- learn the commercial times necessary for the extension service
- guide to the different appointment times when applying single extension strands and extension wefts
- study the quantity of extension hair needed for the different extension hairstyles
- the necessity of hair maintenance appointments

APPOINTMENT TIMES

The hair extension service takes a varied amount of time to perform and it is important to get the timing of appointments right. Incorrect appointment times will affect the profitability of the service.

This service, like all hairdressing services, needs practice to build commercial speed and technique. Work on models and then on clients to gain speed and to perfect the chosen extension application technique.

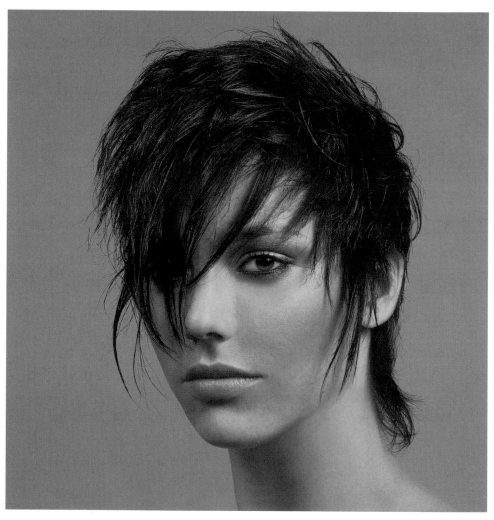

Pierre Balmain, courtesy of Euro Hair Fashion, world licensed manufacturer of Balmain Hair Extensions

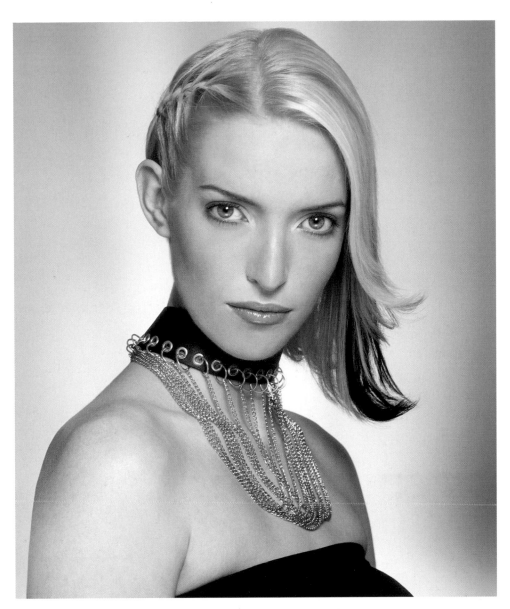

Hair by Aphrodite (Falkirk) and Peter and Bernard (Bathgate), photography Jim Crone

Individual extension strands

It takes one minute to apply one single loose free-flowing extension strand properly. One extension strand weighs approximately one gram. Appointment times and the quantity of hair required for the various extension techniques and hairstyles are shown below.

Hair additions

This hairstyle requires one to fifty extension strands and 1–50 grams of extension hair. It takes 10 minutes to prepare the extension hair before application and 10 minutes to cut, style and blend the extension hair into a natural hairstyle. The hair addition service takes from 30 minutes to 1 hour to complete.

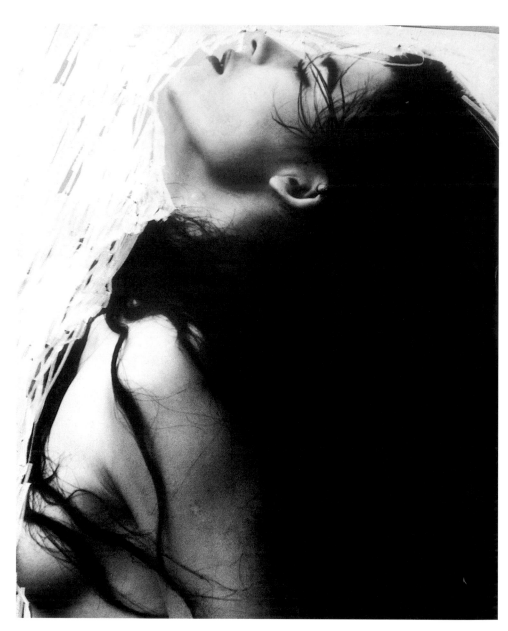

Hair by Jennifer Cheyne

Hair enhancements

In order to achieve this hairstyle use 50–100 extension strands and 50–100 grams of extension hair. It takes 20 minutes to prepare the extension hair before application and 20 minutes to cut, style and blend the extension. The hair enhancement hairstyle takes $1\frac{1}{2}$ to $2\frac{1}{2}$ hours to complete.

Hair extensions

This hairstyle requires 100–250 single extension strands, using 100–250 grams of extension hair. It takes 30 minutes to prepare the extension hair prior to application and 45 minutes to cut and style the extended hairstyle. This service can take 3–$5\frac{1}{2}$ hours to complete.

> **REMEMBER** !
>
> Calculate in the product quantity and the product cost when scheduling hair extension appointment times and therefore the pricing of this service.

The table below outlines the extension appointment times recommended when applying single strands of extensions to create the required hairstyle.

Single strand application

Hairstyle service requirements	Product quantity	Extension hair synthetic fibre and real human hair product weight	Preparing and cutting the extension hair	Time including mixing hair, application, cutting and styling
Hair additions	1–50 extensions	1–50 grams	20 minutes	30 minutes – 1 hour
Hair enhancements	50–100 extensions	50–100 grams	40 minutes	$1\frac{1}{2}$–$2\frac{1}{2}$ hours
Hair extensions	100–250 extensions	100–250 grams	$1\frac{1}{4}$ hours	3–$5\frac{1}{2}$ hours

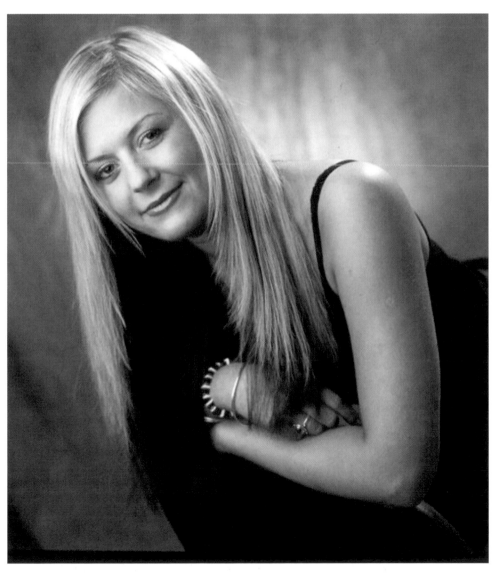

Great Lengths

TOP TIP ✔

Due to the length of time that
this hairstyle takes to complete it
is recommended that two hair
extension practitioners work
together on one client: a trained
stylist and a trained assistant. This
reduces the time it takes to
create the hair alternative
hairstyle.

Hair alternatives

The hair alternative service requires larger quantities of extension hair per individual strand. The larger quantities of extension hair create a texture, such as a dreadlock or a braid. Each loose extension strand weighs 2–3 grams and each texture – such as a dreadlock – takes 3–5 minutes to apply. The hair alternative hairstyle requires 100–250 extension strands. When applying 100 hair extensions into a client's hair at 2–3 grams per extension, use 200–300 grams of extension hair. It takes 30 minutes to prepare the extension hair before application and approximately 30 minutes to cut and style the alternative hairstyle after application. Applying 100 extensions and creating a dreadlock or a braided hair extension hairstyle takes 6–9 hours.

When applying 250 hair alternatives into a client's hairstyle at 2–3 grams per extension, use 500–750 grams of extension hair. It will take 30 minutes to prepare the extension hair prior to application and then approximately 30 minutes to cut and style the hair alternative hairstyle after application. Applying 250 hair alternative extensions into a client's hairstyle can take from $13\frac{1}{2}$–22 hours to complete.

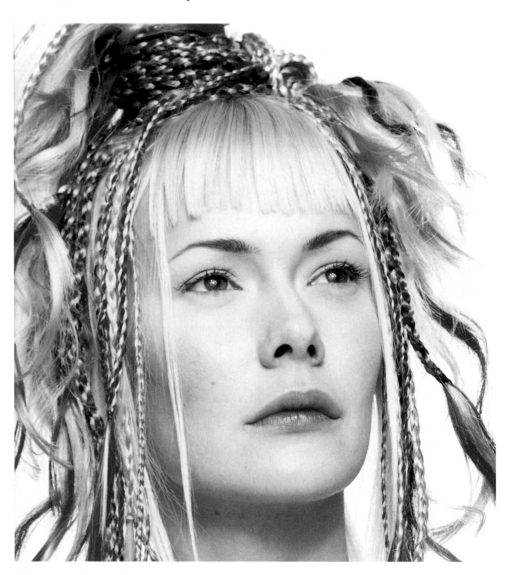

DOME (www.domecosmetics.com)

The table below shows the appointment time necessary when only one practitioner is working on a client.

Single strand and texture application

Hairstyle service requirements	Product quantity	Extension hair synthetic fibre and real hair product weight	Preparing and cutting the extension hair	Time including mixing hair, cutting and styling
Hair alternatives	100 extensions	2–3 grams per extension = 200–300 grams in total	1 hour	6–9 hours
Hair alternatives	250 extensions	2–3 grams per extension = 500–750 grams in total	1 hour	13½–22 hours

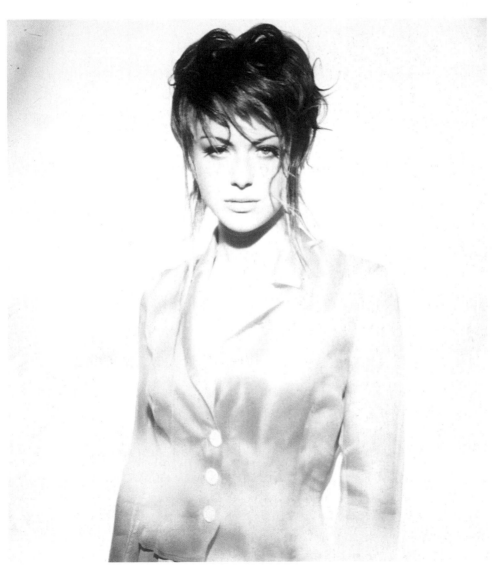

Hair by Jennifer Cheyne

Wefts

The appointment times above have covered the application of individual extension strands. The application of wefts of extension hair takes considerably less time than single extension strands. The use of a cold-fusion system to apply wefts can create hair additions, hair enhancements and hair extensions.

Wefts of hair are applied into a client's hairstyle in rows. It takes approximately 10 minutes to apply one row of wefted hair. It takes 5 minutes to prepare the extension hair before application. The table at the bottom of this page is a guideline to assist in calculating the correct appointment time for this service.

Hair addition

Hairstyles using wefts require 1–2 rows of wefted extension hair and 1–50 grams of hair. It takes 5 minutes to prepare the weft before application and 10 minutes to cut and style into a client's existing hairstyle. Therefore this service takes 25–35 minutes to complete.

Hair enhancement

Hair enhancement hairstyles require 2–4 rows of wefts and 50–100 grams of extension hair. It takes 5 minutes to prepare the extension hair prior to application and 35 minutes to cut and style into a client's existing hairstyle. This service takes 1–1$\frac{1}{2}$ to complete.

Hair extension

Hairstyles require 4–8 rows of wefted extension hair, using 100–250 grams of extension hair. It takes 30 minutes to prepare the extension hair prior to application and 30 minutes to cut and style the extended hairstyle. This service, using wefts takes 1$\frac{1}{2}$–2$\frac{1}{2}$ hours to complete.

Application of wefts

Hairstyle service requirements	No of extension rows	Extension hair synthetic fibre and real human hair product weight	Preparing and cutting the extension hair	Time including mixing hair, cutting and styling
Hair additions	1–2 rows	1–50 grams	15 minutes	25–35 minutes
Hair enhancement	2–4 rows	50–100 grams	40 minutes	1–1$\frac{1}{2}$ hours
Hair extensions	4–8 rows	100–250 grams	1 hour	1$\frac{1}{2}$–2$\frac{1}{2}$ hours

Sewing wefts

When sewing wefts onto a client's hairstyle they are sewn onto a scalp plait or a cornrow. It takes approximately 30 minutes–1 hour to create a scalp plait over a whole head; it takes 5 minutes to prepare the extension hair before application. It then takes 1–2 hours to sew a weft onto a scalp plait and 30 minutes to cut and style the weft into its new hairstyle after application. The table below shows the sewing extension system appointment times. The hairstyle services that are recommended for the sewing system are hair extensions and hair alternatives.

Hair alternatives

Dreadlocks and braids can be bought pre-made on a weft. Scalp plait one continuous row covering the client's whole head. Use 100–250 grams of extension hair.

Sewing wefts

Hairstyle service requirements	No of extension rows	Extension hair synthetic fibre and real human hair product weight	Scalp plaiting preparing, and cutting the extension hair	Time including mixing hair, cutting and styling
Hair extensions	1 continuous row covering the whole head	100–250 grams	1–2 hours	2–3 hours
Hair alternatives	1 continuous row covering the whole head	100–250 grams	1–2 hours	2–3 hours

The above appointment times are guidelines to allocate profitable periods of time for this service. The appointment time depends on the hairstyle discussed with a client during a full consultation.

MAINTENANCE APPOINTMENTS

It is vitally important that extension hairstyles are cared for and maintained during the three months that they are worn. An extension hairstyle does not behave in the same way as natural hair and therefore needs more maintenance.

The type of extension system used will dictate the number of maintenance appointments required. Three different maintenance services are required: the *tidy-up* or *fill-in*, the *styling or re-curling* and the *removal appointment*.

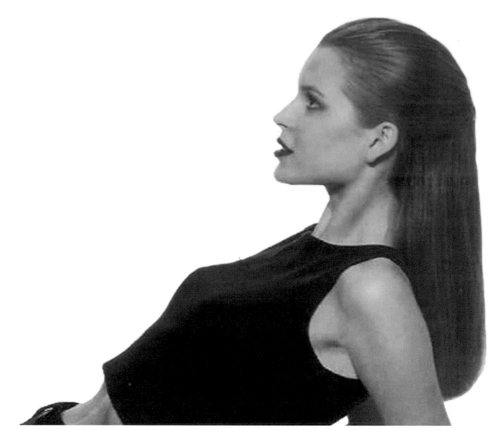

Mane Connection Enhancement System

Tidy-up/fill-in appointments

Clients will need a tidy-up or fill-in appointment half way through the lifetime of the hair extension hairstyle (usually about 4–6 weeks after the extension application). This service includes a shampoo, cut or trim and styling of the extension hair, and natural hair if applicable. Two to ten extensions are lost in a four to six week period of time; the extension hair also moults a little and gaps can appear in the extension hairstyle. Apply some extensions to fill these gaps or replace the extensions that have fallen out. Use 1–20 extensions, which is 1–20 grams of extension hair. A tidy-up appointment takes approximately 1–2 hours.

Styling and re-curling

When wearing wavy or curly fibre hair the wave or curl drops after time and the curl is lost. A styling appointment should be scheduled to re-curl the fibre. This styling or re-curling takes 1–2 hours.

The removal appointment

A removal appointment must be booked three months after extensions have been applied. All extension systems must be removed at the end of three months wear. Every person loses 80–100 hairs per day as natural **hair fall**.

When the client is wearing extensions this loose hair begins to entwine becoming trapped at the root area above the extension bonds or attachment method.

After three months, matting or tangling will occur at the root area between the client's scalp and the bonds that hold the extensions in place. If extensions are left in for more than three months, the tangling becomes difficult to comb out and damage to the natural hair will occur. It takes 1–2 hours to remove extensions.

The following table shows the maintenance appointments, times and product quantities.

Maintenance

Service	Product quantity	Time
Tidy-up or fill-in appointment including a cut or trim	1–20 extensions	1–2 hours
Styling and re-curling		1–2 hours
Removal		1–2 hours

Knowledge review

1 How long does one extension strand take to apply correctly?

2 How many extension strands are applied to create an enhancement hairstyle?

3 How many grams of extension hair are needed to create an alternative extension hairstyle when applying individual strands?

4 When working with wefts, how long does it take to apply one row of wefts using a cold-fusion extension system?

5 How long does it take to prepare a weft of hair before applying it as a hair extension hairstyle?

6 What is another word for a scalp plait?

7 How long does it take to sew a scalp plait over a whole head?

8 How long does a tidy-up appointment take to complete?

9 Why are extensions removed after three months maximum wear?

10 How long does it take to remove extension hairstyles?

chapter 5

CLIENT CONSULTATIONS

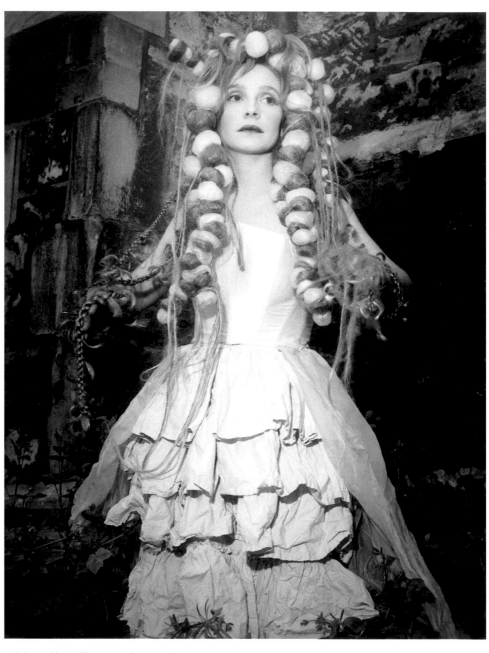

Hair by Jackie McShannon, photography Anders

Learning objectives

- **learn the areas that extensions are placed in on the head**
- **study the different placements of extensions**
- **introduction to the variety of section shapes and sizes of extensions**
- **understand the quantities and length of extension hair to use to create an extension hairstyle**

CLIENT CONSULTATIONS

When introducing the hair extension service into a business, it is essential to conduct thorough client consultations. A client consultation for the hair extension service should take no less than 30 minutes.

Prepare two **client consultation sheets** per client, keep one copy for the customer and one copy for the practitioner. There should be no charge for the consultation as three out of five clients continue with the service after a consultation. A client will not continue with the service after a consultation for several reasons:

- The natural hair is not long or strong enough to hold extensions in place.
- The client's natural **hair texture** is not suitable for the hair extension service.
- The aftercare procedures are inconvenient.
- The price quoted for the service is not within the client's budget.

The hair extension service is the third technical hairdressing service and should be treated as seriously and professionally as other technical services, like colouring and perming. It is therefore important to analyse the condition, strength and suitability of natural hair before applying hair

TOP TIP

To save time, try to arrange to conduct consultations with more than one client at a time.

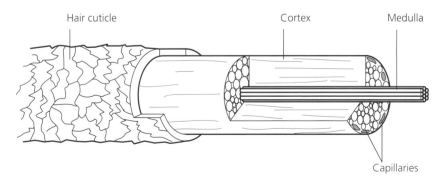

Cross-section of a healthy strand of natural hair

extensions. Analyse the first 4 cm of the natural hair at the root area – this is where all extensions are attached. Decide whether the condition is normal, dry, greasy or broken. If a client has greasy hair, producing excessive sebum so that they have to shampoo their hair every day, then it is not suitable for any extension system. Sebum or natural oils secreted from the hair and scalp will break extension bonds down and will make the natural hair too slippery for the extension bonds to attach. Additionally, if the natural hair in the first 4 cm is broken, it is not suitable for extensions.

Look at the **porosity** of the natural hair in the first 4 cm. If it has been chemically treated, analyse whether the chemical treatment has made the hair weak. If the hair is strong enough to hold the extension bonds in place then go ahead and apply the extensions.

If the first 4 cm is **porous** due to bleaching or relaxing and is weak or broken, it is not suitable for the hair extension service. The mid-lengths and ends of the client's natural hair should be unaffected by the application of extensions, but if it is broken and excessively damaged the friction that can be caused wearing hair extensions can, in extreme cases, result in breakage and hair loss.

Strand test

Apply four–six extension strands in different areas over the client's head and schedule a **strand test** check appointment 7–14 days later. During the appointment look at the test strands; check that the natural hair has held the extension without any breakage. Check the natural hair has not been pulled out of the scalp. Check for scalp irritation or a rash on the scalp. Remove the test strand, check that there are not excessive amounts of natural hair trapped in the extension bond. Check that the client has managed to shampoo, condition and style the extension hair at home.

Skin sensitivity test

A strand test performs two functions: to check the strength of the client's natural hair before applying extensions and to see whether the client is sensitive to the products used.

Some clients have severe allergies (e.g. to peanuts, seafood, chicken or eggs) that can cause an anaphylactic shock. The hot melt and cold-fusion adhesives are prepared using secret formulas that are patented to the product companies. Often the ingredients are not advertised. Over the 23 years that hair extensions have been on the marketplace, on very rare occasions, clients have suffered allergic reactions to the extension hair, adhesives or aftercare products.

Before conducting a skin sensitivity test on a client who suffers from **allergies** ensure they are aware of the potential danger and are prepared with medication to deal with a potential hazard. *This is absolutely vital and can be a matter of life or death for some clients.*

Most clients who suffer from anaphylactic shock have medication with them to deal with this condition.

REMEMBER

Always apply a strand and skin sensitivity test to check the **tensile strength** of natural hair and potential skin sensitivities before applying extensions.

REMEMBER

If you would not be prepared to tint, bleach or perm a client's hair then you must not apply extensions to that client's hair.

HEALTH AND SAFETY

During a consultation, ask clients whether they suffer from any allergies or have any allergic reaction that would result in an anaphylactic shock.

CONTRA-INDICATIONS OF THE HAIR EXTENSION SERVICE

During consultation ascertain whether a client has any medical or physical conditions that may prevent the application of the hair extension service. These conditions are called **contra-indications**. If a client suffers from any of the following contra-indications do not apply extensions.

- Treatments for hair fall, alopecia, psoriasis or eczema on their head: the hair extension service will aggravate skin conditions
- Infestations such as head lice or the nit eggs on natural hair
- Breakage through the first 4 cm of their hair at the root area
- Excessively greasy hair – greasy hair will break bonds down and extensions will slide out
- Do not apply extensions on a client who is pregnant or within 6 months of childbirth. Pregnancy can increase hair fall conditions and an extension hairstyle can make the hair fall worse. The client may think that the extensions have caused the hair fall rather than it being a natural condition brought about by childbirth
- Do not apply extensions on any client who is taking treatment for cancer. Do not apply extensions into any client's hair within 6 months after cancer treatment has been completed. Medication for cancer sadly can make hair fall out completely and extensions will speed up this process.

> **TOP TIP**
>
> Infestations must be cleared completely before applying the hair extension service.

DECIDING ON THE EXTENSION HAIRSTYLE

During consultation establish the extension hairstyle required. Take notes when the client is describing exactly what hairstyle they are looking for. Discuss the differences between real extension hair, fibre extension hair, weaves, wefts, pre-bonded hair extensions, fashion braids, fashion textures and so on. Guide and recommend clients to choose the correct extension hair for their hair texture, structure and hairstyle.

Hair texture

Decide which extension hair structure and texture will be suitable for the desired result.

> **REMEMBER** !
>
> Match the texture and structure of extension hair to the client's natural hair. For example, if a client has straight fine natural hair, use straight European extension hair or straight fibre extension hair to create their hair extension hairstyle. Natural hair must be coloured, straightened or permed before applying extensions because the extension hair used matches the new structure or colour of the natural hair.

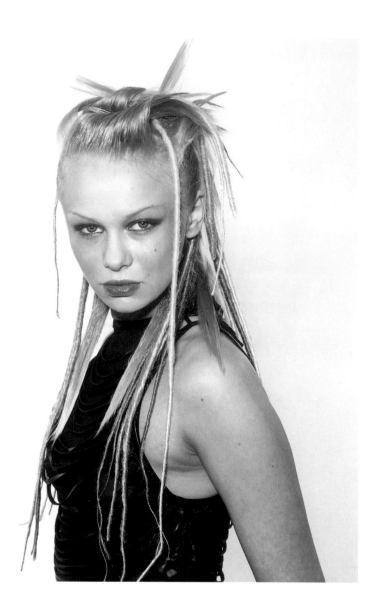

Hair by Jason Smith

Hair length

The next area to cover during a consultation is the extension hair length that the client wants – the price of extension hair increases depending on the length of the hair that is to be used.

> **REMEMBER** !
>
> When creating a natural-looking extension hairstyle never more than double the length of the client's existing hairstyle. If you do so, the extension hairstyle will not blend and will not look natural and the extension hair will place unnecessary strain on the hair shaft, causing hair loss.

Analyse the client's natural **hair length and density** to ensure that it is a suitable length for wearing an extension hairstyle. The required length will depend on the type of extension hairstyle the client is looking for.

Hair additions

Natural hair must be a minimum of $7\frac{1}{2}$ cm long to be able to wear a hair addition hairstyle. The reason for this is that the natural hair has to be long enough to cover any bonds or attachments that hold an extension hair strand in place.

Hair enhancements

To achieve this hairstyle the natural hair must be a minimum of 13 cm long.

Hair extensions

When creating an extended hairstyle, the natural hair must be a minimum of $15\frac{1}{2}$ cm long. This is because the client's natural hair must be long enough to cover the bonds that attach the extensions in place. It must also be long enough and strong enough to hold the extensions in place for up to three months' wear.

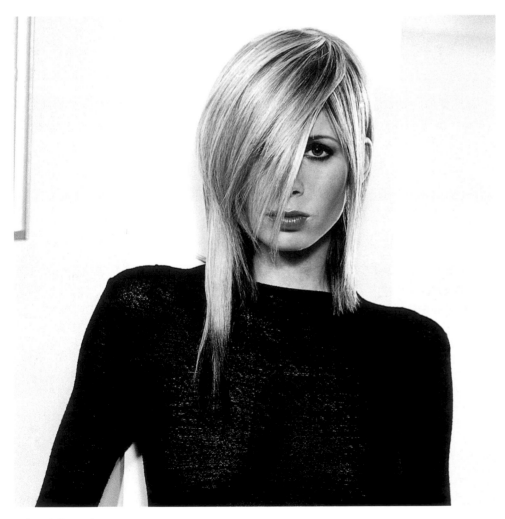

Jack Melville at Cheynes

Hair alternatives

When applying a hair alternative hairstyle the hair must be the minimum of $7\frac{1}{2}$ cm long, as with hair additions. It is not as important with hair alternatives to hide the bonds. What is important is that you have enough length of hair to braid or secure the extensions. If the client's hair is $7\frac{1}{2}$ cm long, you should only take these extensions to 15 cm long.

Again, if you are in doubt as to whether the client's natural hair is long enough and strong enough to wear a hair addition, enhancement, extension or alternatives hairstyle, do a strand test and check it in 7–14 days' time. Often, during the consultation, after discovering exactly what hairstyle the client is looking for their natural hair is too short to cover the extension hair; therefore the hairstyle won't blend and it will not look like a natural hairstyle. You will need to advise your clients to let their hair grow and to come back in 3–9 months' time. Natural hair grows a quarter to a half an inch ($\frac{1}{2}$–1 cm) a month as an average, so it is easy to calculate how much longer it will need to be. The client must not cut their hair – not even to have it trimmed or thinned out – during this period.

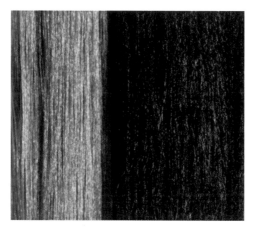
Silky straight real hair   American Dream

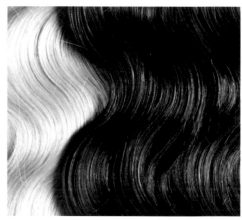
Soft wave real hair   American Dream

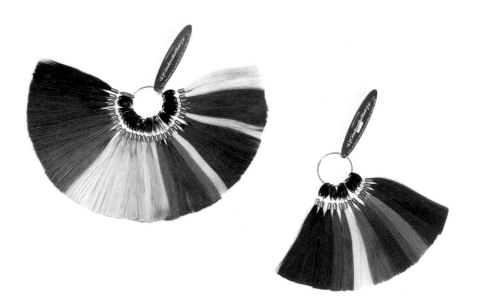
Colour rings   Cinderella

Hair colour

Select extension hair colours that are needed to create the client's desired hairstyle. Use a colour ring containing the swatches of extension hair in the colours available from the product company. Place the colour ring up to the client's real hair and select the extension hair colour that matches the client's natural hair colour. Each extension hair packet is numbered and each number represents a colour – make a note of the number of the correct colour. This will help to order the hair for your client's particular hairstyle.

Aftercare requirements

During the consultation discuss the aftercare requirements for the specific hair extension hairstyle. The products needed in stock ready for resale include clarifying shampoos, reconstructive conditioners, leave-in conditioners, pH-balanced sprays, de-tangling sprays and soft bristle brushes. Discuss the specific home care requirements for the extension hairstyle; these products must be used throughout the three-month duration of the extension hairstyle.

Let the client know how long the hair extension hairstyle will take to apply. Do this by estimating how much extension hair will be used.

Order the same quantity of extension hair as the quantity of natural hair on the head. Using the table in the appointments time section and working on the principle that it takes 1 minute to apply 1 extension and 10 minutes to apply 1 wefted row of extensions, calculate how long the extension appointment is going to take. Write the estimated time on your consultation sheet.

TOP TIP

Take hold of the client's hair in a pony tail and feel the quantity of natural hair being held. When applying extension hairstyles only double the thickness of the natural hair. This will ensure that the extension hairstyle looks and feels authentic.

MAINTENANCE APPOINTMENTS

At this point in the consultation, cover the specific **maintenance appointments** needed. These appointments are to be booked at two-week intervals if styling or re-curling extension hair. Four-week appointments are scheduled for sewn and cold-fusion systems. Six-week appointments are scheduled for hot systems. Schedule the removal appointment – the maximum time to wear an extension hairstyle is 12 weeks.

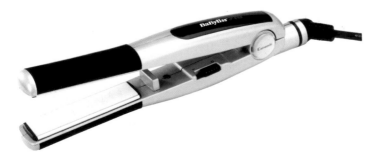

Straightening irons   BaByliss

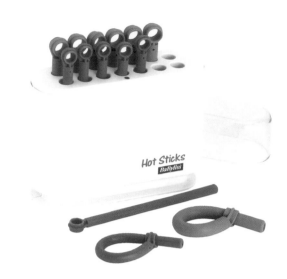

Heated sticks   BaByliss

Deposits

Discuss the cost of the desired hair extension hairstyle then book the appointment date and time and take a **non-refundable deposit**. The balance is to be paid on completion of the appointment. A deposit assures a client that a practitioner will be available to perform the hair extension hairstyle discussed. Additionally the deposit will cover lost revenue if a client does not turn up for the appointment. The client must be fully aware that the deposit is non-refundable. This means that if they cancel or move their appointment, they can move their deposit, but the deposit will not be refunded. You must give a receipt for a non-refundable deposit. Take a deposit after all strand and skin sensitivity tests have been completed.

Declaration and agreement

Ensure clients understand that it is essential to follow all aftercare instructions and stylist's advice during the lifetime of the hair extension hairstyle. Ensure the strand test and skin sensitivity test check appointment is scheduled in 7–14 days. After checking the test go ahead and book the hair extension appointment.

Colouring

The strand test period of 7–14 days between the initial consultation and the extension application allows enough time to colour the client's hair if required. This chemical colour work, if the hair is strong enough, should be done prior to the application of the hair extension service. Match the colour of the extension hair to the client's natural hair colour that you have tinted before ordering the fibre or real extension hair. File the client consultation form safely.

An example of a client consultation form appears opposite.

CLIENT CONSULTATION FORM

Client name.. Tel ....

<u>Natural hair analysis:</u> normal.. dry.................................. greasy .... broken ....

<u>Natural hair porosity:</u> virgin................................... chemically treated .... bleached..................

<u>Check the contraindications of hair extensions – Do a strand and skin sensitivity test</u>

<u>Extension hairstyle required</u>

Additions .... Enhancements .... Extensions......................... Alternatives .... Other....................

Additional style notes ....

<u>Client's natural hair length:</u>   7.5 cm .... 13 cm .... 15.5 cm...............................

<u>Extension hair required:</u>   Asian hair ..... European hair .... Fibre hair ...Wefts ..... Pre-bonded hair .... Fashion braids ....

<u>Extension hair texture required:</u>   Straight............. Soft wave............. Deep wave............ Spiral curl .... Other ....

<u>Extension hair length required:</u>

10"/20 cm .... 12"/24 cm .... 14"/28 cm .... 16"/32 cm .... 18"/36 cm .... 20"/40 cm .... 24"/48 cm or more ....

<u>Extension hair colours selected:</u> ....

<u>Client aftercare requirements</u>

Shampoo ... Reconstruct conditioner ... Leave-in conditioner ... pH-balanced spray ... De-tangle spray ... Soft brush ...

<u>Appointment time</u>

30 mins .... 1 hour .... 2 hours .... 3 hours .... 4 hours .... 5 hours .... 6 hours .... More than six hours .....

<u>Maintenance appointments</u>

Tidy-up   every 2 weeks .... 4 weeks .... 6 weeks ....

Styling or re-curling   every 2 weeks .... 4 weeks .... 6 weeks ....

Removal   2 weeks .... 4 weeks .... 6 weeks .... 8 weeks .... 10 weeks .... 12 weeks ....

Total price .... 50% Deposit .... Balance to pay .... Appointment date .... Time ....

<u>All deposits are non-refundable</u> It is essential to follow all aftercare instructions and stylist advice during the lifetime of a hair extension hairstyle (see aftercare sheet). In order to maintain extension hairstyles client must have them serviced at the salon at regular intervals recommended by their stylist. All hair extension systems must be removed from natural hair at the end of three months' wear.

I agree to abide by the terms and conditions of my stylist recommendations for my hair extension hairstyle.

Signed by client.. Signed by stylist .... Date...................................

Knowledge review

1 When analysing the natural hair's condition and porosity what area of the hair are you checking and why?

2 Why should a strand test be taken before applying hair extensions?

3 What does contra-indication mean?

4 How long should natural hair be to apply:

- hair additions

- hair enhancements

- hair extensions

- hair alternatives

Why?

5 When extending hair, why can you only double the length of the natural hair?

6 When adding extensions, why can you only double the thickness of the natural hair?

7 Explain what the three maintenance appointments are and how long they take to complete.

8 Why is it important to take a non-refundable deposit when a client has booked an extension appointment?

9 When should chemical colours be applied before applying extensions?

10 Where do you file consultation forms or record cards?

chapter 6

THE HAIR

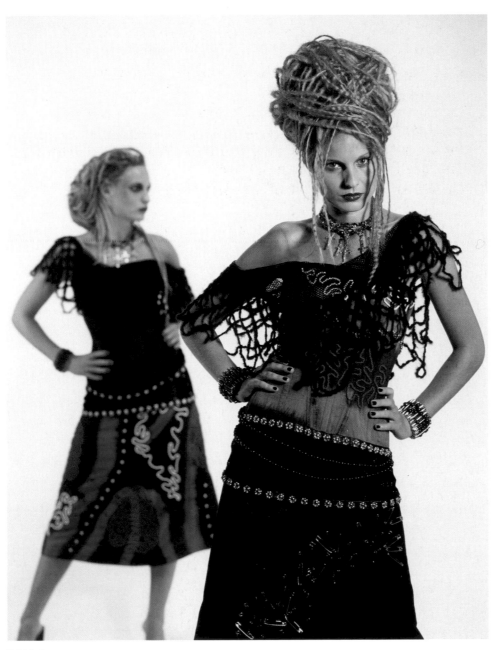

Patrick Cameron

- **how chemical processes can be applied before and during the hair extension service**
- **how to pre-cut natural hair before applying extensions**
- **cleanse and condition natural hair before application of extensions**
- **select extension hair colours**
- **understand how to blend real and fibre hair**
- **mixing and blending extension hair using the colour formula**

PREPARING THE NATURAL HAIR BEFORE APPLYING A HAIR EXTENSION SERVICE

TOP TIP

You cannot make curly hair straight or straight hair curly by simply adding extension hair.

Preparing the natural hair is very important, because it becomes the base that enables the completed extension hairstyle to look authentic. When working on natural curly hair apply wavy or curly extension hair. When working on natural straight hair apply straight extension hair. *Perform all chemical treatments such as perming, straightening or colour treatments prior to applying hair extensions.* Extension hair must match the texture of the natural hair.

Chemical processes

REMEMBER

If the colour and texture of the extension hair does not match the natural hair, the extension hair will not blend with the new style. There will be a divide between the two hair types and the extension hairstyle will appear false and be unattractive.

Allow 1–2 days between performing a chemical process and applying extensions. After these procedures the practitioner can order the correct colour and texture of extension hair.

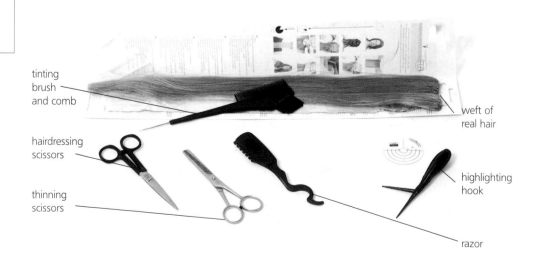

tinting brush and comb

weft of real hair

hairdressing scissors

highlighting hook

thinning scissors

razor

The period of time left between a chemical process on natural hair and the extension application is important because the chemical products will affect the bonds that attach the extension hair.

Analyse the natural hair after a chemical process to ensure that it is still strong enough to hold the extension hair in place. As with other chemical processes, the treatment can weaken the hair to such a degree that it will not hold the extension hairstyle in place, so complete a strand test before extension application.

Perming and colouring whilst wearing an extension hairstyle

Chemical processes must be applied carefully throughout the duration of the extension hairstyle. Perming is not recommended while wearing hair extensions. Most perms will last for three months, so perm natural hair before applying extensions and after removing extensions.

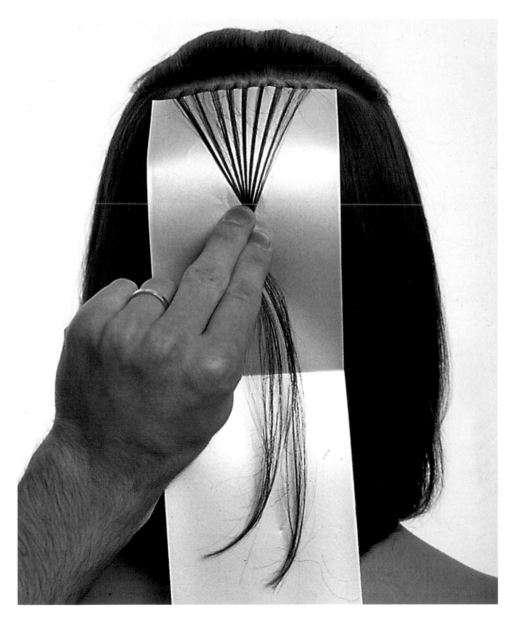

Mahogany

Apply extension strand tests after perming or colouring natural hair to check the strength and durability of the newly chemically treated hair.

During the three months that hair extensions are worn, root **regrowth application** of colour on the hairline, parting and around the crown of natural hair can be applied. Do not touch up the root regrowth of natural hair through the interior of the hairstyle. Avoid applying permanent colour on the extension bonds or attachments as the chemical colour could weaken the bonds and they will crumble and fall out.

Highlights

Use foils to highlight the hairline, parting and crown area of natural hair. When using a foil highlighting process avoid the interior of the extension hairstyle as it is impossible to get close enough to the root area to colour the regrowth.

COLOURING REAL EXTENSION HAIR

Do not use a permanent colour or perm on extension hair – the chemical processes will give an unpredictable result. This is because extension hair has undergone several chemical processes.

Use semi-permanent or quasi-colours on the extension hair to the maximum peroxide strength of 4 per cent, this will add tone or depth to the extension colour. Do not attempt to lighten extension hair, as lightening products will chemically over-process the extension hair, leaving it too damaged to use.

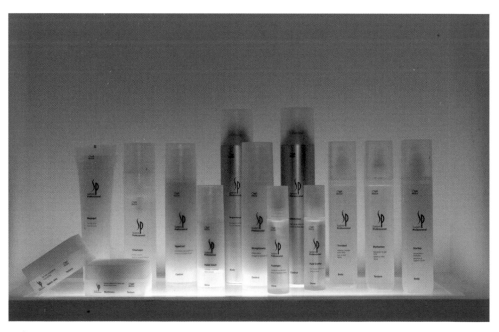

Wella

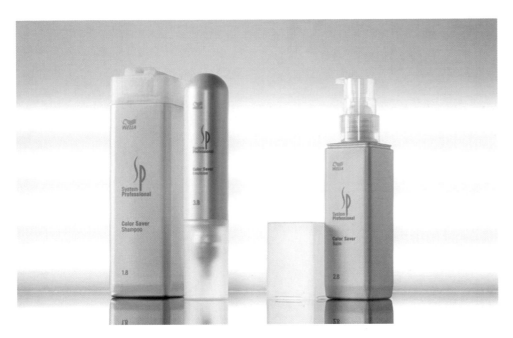

Wella

CUTTING THE NATURAL HAIR

Natural hair must be at certain minimum lengths to create the various hair extension hairstyles. The natural hairstyle may need to be cut prior to applying extensions into the hair. If your client is wearing a solid straight blunt haircut as their natural hairstyle, the straight blunt line must be removed prior to creating an extended (longer) hairstyle. If the blunt line is kept in and extensions are applied, the blunt line will protrude through the extension hairstyle and the hairstyle will not look natural because there will be an obvious divide between the existing hairstyle and the new extension hairstyle.

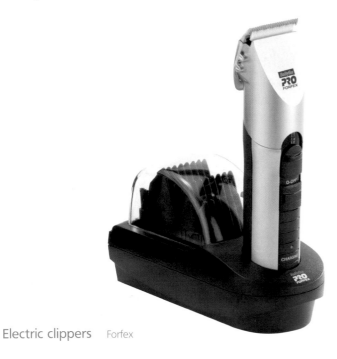

Electric clippers   Forfex

To remove blunt cut lines from the natural hair, the extension practitioner will need to use either tapering scissors, thinning scissors or a razor and, in some cases, a combination of all three tools. The ends of the natural hairstyle must be tapered or thinned so that once the extension hair has been applied there is no demarcation line between the natural and extension hairstyle.

CLEANSING THE NATURAL HAIR

Natural hair must be clean before applying hair extensions. Shampoo with a clarifying shampoo prior to the application. Clarifying shampoos remove sebum, oil, grease, styling products, pollution, chlorine or any other unseen residues that may be deposited on the client's natural hair. These residues must be removed as they can affect the adhesion of the polymer resins. If the natural hair has been chemically treated – i.e. permed or coloured – prior to extension application, lightly condition the ends of the natural hair, otherwise do not apply a conditioner as it can form a barrier affecting the adhesion of resin bonds.

Once shampooed and conditioned, natural hair must be dried thoroughly before applying the extensions. Natural hair is porous (it absorbs water). When it has absorbed water the hair shaft swells and when it dries it shrinks.

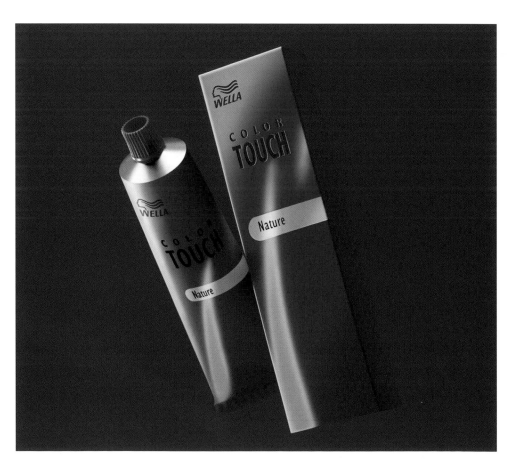

Wella

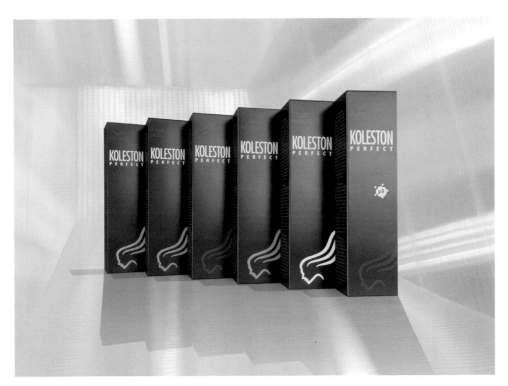

Wella

If applying an extension bond on damp hair or hair that contains water, when it dries it will shrink and this causes the bond to loosen and fall out of the hair.

Blow-dry the natural hair into style, arranging partings in place prior to extension application.

HAIR PREPARATION CHECKLIST

- Ensure that the client's natural hair length is the minimum required for attaching extensions and to achieve the target hairstyle.

- Shampoo the client's hair in a clarifying shampoo to remove any deposits or impurities that may affect the bonds holding the extensions in place.

- Lightly condition the client's natural hair at the mid-lengths and ends only. Do not apply conditioner on the root area. Conditioner should only be used if the natural hair has undergone a technical chemical process.

- Using a razor, tapering or thinning scissors, thin, graduate or taper the ends (the last 2–4 cm of the client's natural hair) to reduce any solid weight lines, blunt straight lines or thick ends in the natural hair. This allows the extension hair and the natural hair to blend together.

- Dry the hair into the hairstyle that the client requires. Make sure it has been dried thoroughly before applying extensions.

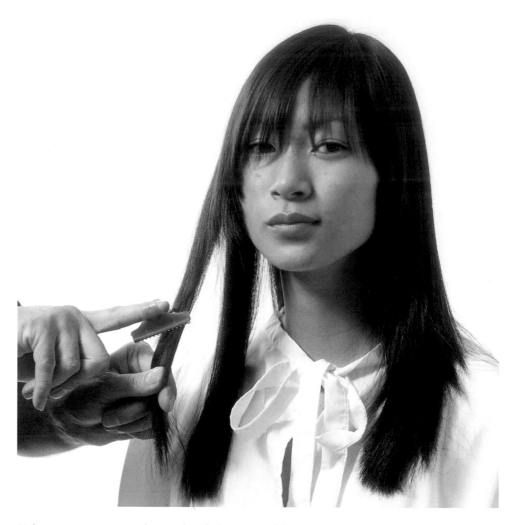

Using a razor, taper the ends of the natural hair to soften the perimeter

PREPARING THE EXTENSION HAIR BEFORE APPLYING A HAIR EXTENSION SERVICE

Mixing and blending extension hair

Mixing and blending extension hair is the process that the extension practitioner uses to create an extension hair colour to match the client's natural hair colour or create a pre-agreed colour application, such as a tonal or highlighted colour.

Selecting extension hair colour

The method of selecting extension hair colour is exactly the same with real and fibre extension hair. Using a **colour ring** place it next to the natural hair and find the swatch of hair colour that matches the natural hair colour as closely as possible. Always match to the mid-lengths and ends of the client's natural hair, not the root area. The root area is darker than the mid-lengths and ends.

The first colour to select is called the **base** or **first colour**. Identify a second colour nearest to the colour of the natural hair. This is called the **major tone** or **second colour**. Look closely for a third colour that matches the hue or the glint of the natural hair colour. (Sometimes you will not find a third colour in the client's hair.) Look for tiny strands of colour, such as a percentage of white hair. This is called the **minor tone** or **third colour**.

After identifying the three colours follow the formula to mix and blend extension hair to match natural hair colour. The formula follows a principle very similar to mixing tints when adding in mix tones.

> **REMEMBER !**
>
> This formula is merely a guideline as matching hair is a visual process.

MIXING FORMULA FOR EXTENSION HAIR

- Mixing equal quantities of two extension hair colours together will change the base colour. For example, mixing 10 grams of light brown with 10 grams of dark brown will create a new base colour, which will be a mid-brown that sits exactly between the light and dark brown.

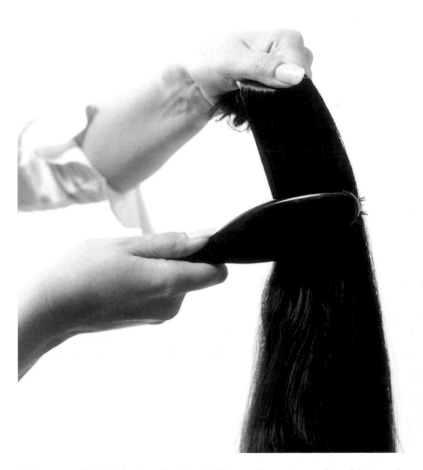

Using a soft-bristle brush, blend fibre colours together (shown here with soft wave fibre hair)

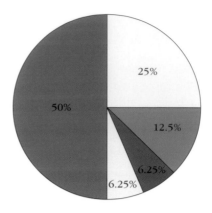

- Mixing a quarter (25 per cent) of a second colour to a first colour will lighten or darken the first colour. For example, $2^1/_2$ grams of blonde with 10 grams of light brown will lighten the light brown by 1–2 shades.

- Mixing one eighth (12.5 per cent) of a second colour to a first colour will give the first colour a strong tone, very similar to the result when a semi-permanent colour is used on natural hair. For example, add 1.75 grams of a burgundy to 10 grams of a light brown. It will give a warm red tone to the light brown.

- Mixing one sixteenth (6.25 per cent) of a second colour to the first colour will give the first colour a hue or glint of colour. For example, add 1 gram of white to 16 grams of light brown. The light brown hair will appear to have some tiny strands of grey hair mixed in with it.

ORDERING THE EXTENSION HAIR

Order the quantities of extension hair required for the hairstyle. Order the extension hair in the correct texture and length.

Each colour ring has swatches of hair in the various colours that the product company supplies. Each extension hair colour has a number allocated to it. This number does not match the international colour coding system used for chemical colours and tints. Rather, it is a stock code that the manufacturers use to differentiate between the extension hair colours. Place orders using the number and describe the colour required.

When the hair arrives

Real hair may be ordered in bulk, which means it is loose with a band tied at one end. This banded end is the root end and it is absolutely vital to keep real extension hair root point correct. When real extension hair is ordered on a weft, the root end is at the sewn wefted end.

Fibre hair will arrive in packets, an elastic band will be on the end of the fibre holding it together to prevent tangling. Fibre does not need to be kept root point correct as fibre does not have a directional cuticle layer.

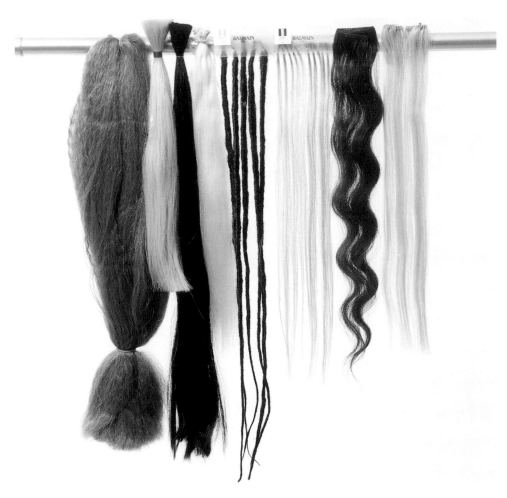

From left to right, jumbo fibre hair, bulk real hair (two bunches), pre-bonded real hair, pre-made dreadlocks, pre-bonded real hair, machine sewn real hair weft, hand sewn real hair weft

MIXING AND BLENDING REAL EXTENSION HAIR

Mixing and blending real extension hair is a quick and simple process. Use a mixing mat.

Place one half of the mixing mat on a work surface with the metal teeth facing upwards. Following the mixing formula place the first, second and third colours onto the teeth of the mixing mat. Place the root ends together with the root ends facing you and the tips travelling away from you. Put the first colour into the teeth of the mixing mat and layer the second colour on top of the first colour. Take the second half of the mixing mat, place it on top of the real hair with the teeth facing downwards. Press the mats firmly together to trap the real hair into this mat. This holds the real hair in place root point correct. Once the extension colours are sandwiched together in the mixing mat, simply pinch a piece of the extension hair, approximately 1 gram in weight or the size of a highlight, and draw it out of the mixing mat between thumb and forefinger. As the real hair draws through the teeth of the mixing mat the colours will blend together.

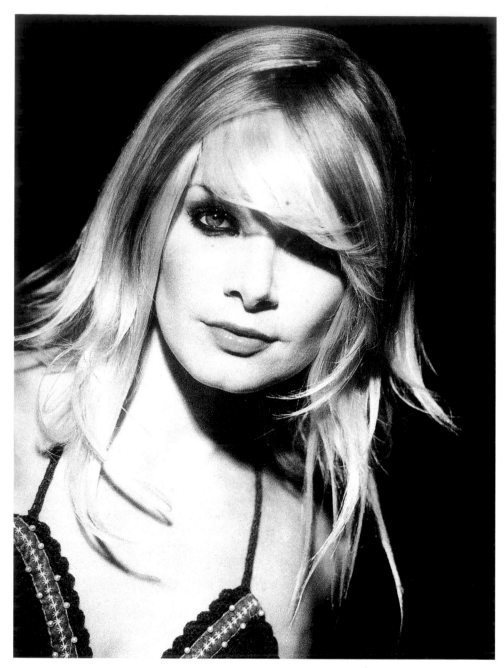

Hair by Jennifer Cheyne

MIXING AND BLENDING FIBRE EXTENSION HAIR

When the fibre hair arrives

Take it out of its packet and cut off the elastic bands at the end of the fibre. These prevent the hair from tangling and are placed there to assist in packaging, storing and transporting. Using the mixing formula divide the fibre into manageable quantities, place colours selected on top of each other.

Hold the fibre hair in its centre. Do not hold it at the end because it could fall onto the floor.

Blending fibre hair

There are two blending techniques used with fibre hair, depending on the colour effect required. These are **bulk blending** (or **mega-mixing**) and **block blending**.

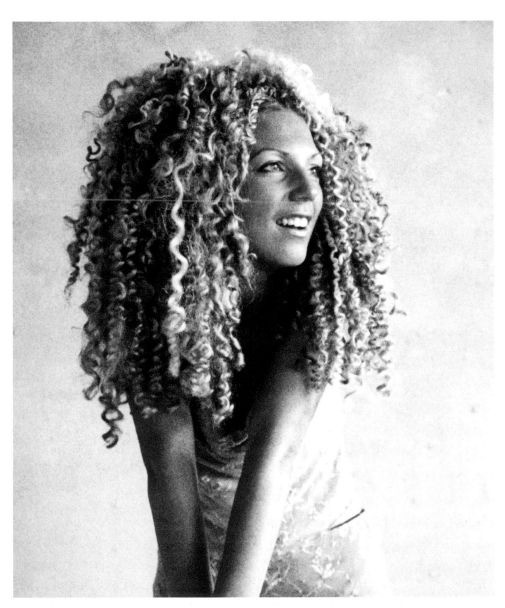

Hair by Jackie McShannon, photography Irvine Miskell-Reid

Bulk blending/mega-mixing

After selecting the quantities of the first, second and third colours, simply place them together, keeping the ends of the fibre hair together to prevent uneven lengths. Hold the fibre hair in its centre and lightly spray the fibre with a de-tangling conditioning spray. This will help to de-tangle the fibre while blending. Using a soft bristle brush, brush the synthetic fibre hair colours together. Start brushing from the ends of the fibre, work towards the centre and continue to brush and blend using a soft bristle brush until all the colours have mixed together. When the fibre is blended, place it up to the natural hair, matching to the mid-lengths and ends. When fibre matches, proceed with the extension application.

Block blending

This technique is used to create a **block colour**, highlights or a streaky colour effect. First select a base colour by matching the colour swatch next to the natural colour, matching to the mid-lengths and ends. Take a contrasting second colour, and place the quantity of second colour on top of the first colour, holding the extension hair in the centre. Divide the extension hair in half, then place the two halves one on top of the other and continue to subdivide four or five times. Do not brush the hair when creating a block colour. The result will be a highlighted or streaked effect.

Knowledge review

1 Why should natural hair be chemically treated before applying extensions?

2 What area of the head can be chemically treated when wearing extensions?

3 What cutting techniques should be used on natural hair before applying extensions?

4 Why should natural hair be clean and dry before extension application?

5 What part of the natural hair should be matched to the extension hair?

6 What do the first, second and third colours represent?

7 What percentage of a second colour should be added to the first colour to lighten or darken the first colour?

8 Why must real extension hair be mixed root point correct?

9 Describe how fibre is blended together.

10 What are bulk blending and block blending?

chapter 7

PLANNING THE APPLICATION OF AN EXTENSION HAIRSTYLE

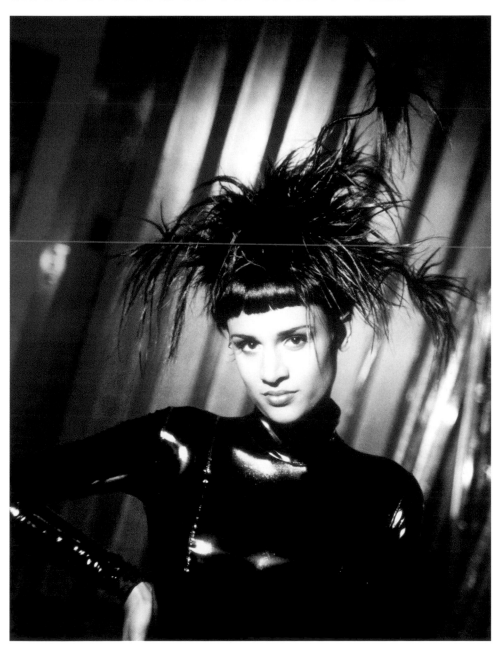

Hair by Jennifer Cheyne

- learn the areas that extensions are placed in on the head
- study the different placements of extensions
- introduction to the variety of section shapes and sizes of extensions
- understand the quantities and length of extension hair to use to create an extension hairstyle

THE AREA SECTIONS OF THE NATURAL HAIR

When planning the application of a hair extension hairstyle first understand the different areas of the head where extensions are applied. There are six areas:

Area 1 The nape area (under the occipital bone)

Area 2 The occipital bone to crown on the back of the head

Area 3 The temple area on the left-hand side

Area 4 The temple area on the right-hand side

Area 5 The recession area on the left-hand side

Area 6 The recession area on the right-hand side.

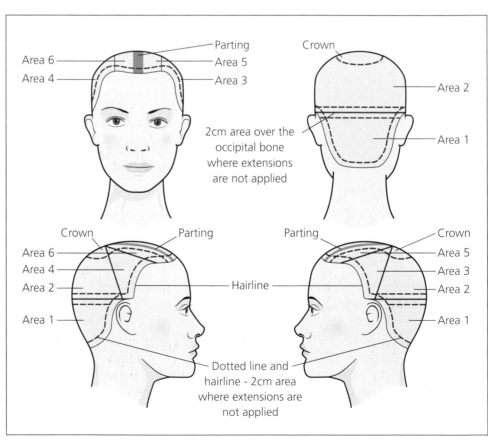

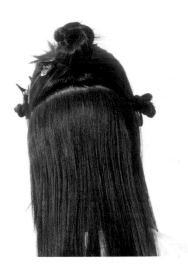

Areas 1 and 2
Hair by Theresa Bullock

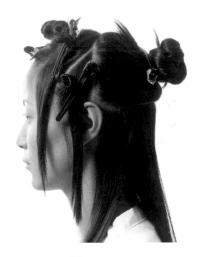

Areas 1, 2, 3 and 5
Hair by Theresa Bullock

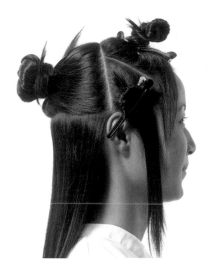

Showing areas 4 and 6
Hair by Theresa Bullock

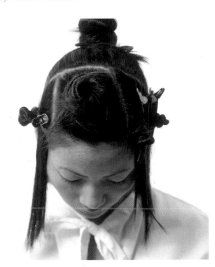

Showing areas 5 and 6
Hair by Theresa Bullock

Extensions are placed in rows throughout the hairstyle and these rows are placed one on top of the other in a brickwork fashion.

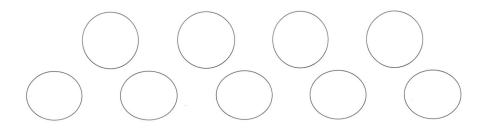

When creating natural-looking hair extension hairstyles place extensions 2 cm inside the hairline, 2 cm away from the parting and the crown, and 2 cm above or below the occipital bone (this is the bone that protrudes from the back of the head just above the nape section). Work extensions in the interior of the natural hairstyle. A 1–2 cm section of natural hair is left out in between each row of extensions.

TOP TIP

Extensions are not applied on the hairline, a parting, near the crown or the occipital bone. If applied on the hairline, parting or crown the bonds that attach the extensions become visible. If applied on the occipital bone, the extensions will protrude through the hairstyle and either the hairstyle shape becomes distorted or the bonds become visible.

PLACEMENT OF EXTENSIONS

There are five **extension placements**:

1 Solid or continuous row of extensions A solid placement of extensions is where a practitioner puts one extension right next to another in a solid row.

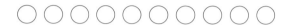

A solid row placement gives a blanket or sheet of hair and provides bulk and thickness. Use solid rows when lengthening natural hair or when complete coverage is required to overtake a natural hairstyle.

2 Closely scattered placement This placement involves placing one extension next to another in a row, leaving a $^1/_4$–$^1/_2$ cm gap of natural hair between.

$$X-X-X-X-X-X-X-X-X$$

This placement gives root lift, volume and thickness. It blends extension hair in with the client's natural hair and lengthens the hairstyle. A closely scattered placement is used when movement and direction are required.

3 Scattered placement A practitioner places one extension next to another in a row leaving a $^1/_2$–1 cm gap in between.

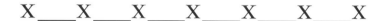

A scattered placement is used to create highlights or lowlights. It also blends natural hair with extension hair and adds body.

4 Visual placement Used when the practitioner examines completed extension hairstyles and places small extensions where gaps appear in the style or where blending is required.

5 Weft placement This is relevant when the practitioner is applying wefts. These are either attached to the client's hair with a cold-fusion gum or sewn onto a scalp plait. They are placed in continuous rows. A weft placement either overrides the existing hairstyle or is incorporated into the interior of the client's hairstyle and can only achieve solid placement. This placement works most successfully on African-Caribbean hairstyles. However, wefts can also be used in solid rows to achieve extension hairstyles on Caucasian, Asian and Oriental hair.

EXTENSION SHAPES AND SIZES

Extensions are applied into natural hair on different natural hair section shapes: squares, triangles or rectangles. The most common sections taken are square. The sections are applied in different extension sizes that depend on the extension system chosen.

Section sizes and shapes

Square sections

Sections half a centimentre square are the most widely used extension size because they enable the practitioner to create an extension hairstyle where the attachments are undetectable. This is because the single loose extension strands and the bonds that attach them are small. To apply a small extension, take a ¹/₂ cm square section of natural hair and using the same quantity of extension hair as there is natural hair in that section, attach the extension at the root area.

Pierre Balmain, courtesy of Euro Hair Fashion, world licensed manufacturer of Balmain Hair Extensions

The extension is attached using a bond. The bond created on this quantity of extension hair should be the same size and shape as a grain of rice. The top of the bond must be placed at the base of the $\frac{1}{2}$ cm square section of natural hair, $\frac{1}{2}$ cm away from the scalp. Placing the bond away from the scalp ensures that the loose extension strand can move without causing unnecessary strain on the natural hair or the hair shaft.

Sections, 1 cm square, using equal amounts of extension and natural hair are used mainly for the braiding systems as a larger circumference of natural hair is required for this technique. Tensioning is a very important consideration when braiding extension hair into natural hair.

African-Caribbean hair is generally quite curly so tensioning when braiding can be tight because the natural curly hair will loosen after a couple of hours, allowing the extension to sit slightly away from the scalp.

Caucasian, Asian and Oriental hair is generally straight. Tensioning when braiding must be firm but not tight as the natural hair will not loosen the braid at the root area. If it is too tight it will pull at the hair shaft causing tension spots, possible breakage and alopecia. Ensure that braids are applied $\frac{1}{2}$–1 cm away from the scalp when working on these hair types to prevent tension problems.

Sections 2 cm square are required when applying hair alternatives such as dreadlocks. A greater quantity of natural hair is required to hold the textured extension without putting any strain on the natural hair.

Triangular sections

Triangular sections come in two sizes: either $\frac{1}{2}$ cm or 1 cm wide. They can be used when working near the parting or crown to help blend the extensions into the natural hairstyle.

Rectangular sections

Rectangular sections are made in two sizes: $\frac{1}{2}$ cm wide $\times$ 1 cm deep or 1 cm wide $\times$ 2 cm deep. They are suitable for clients with curly or African-Caribbean hair and, in some circumstances, for clients with very thick hair. When extensions are applied to these hair types, they can create excessive bulk at the root area. The rectangular section condenses the root area, reducing this bulk to prevent a distorted or misshapen hairstyle. The bond of the extension, braid or extension application that you are working with is to be placed at the base of the rectangular section. Rectangular sections can also be used when applying hair alternative textures, such as dreadlocks.

TOP TIP

Remove the points of the triangle before use. This is because the points take most of the pressure and can break, especially on finer hair.

Choosing size and shape of section

A ½ cm square section of natural hair is taken. The same amount of extension hair is drawn to the quantity of extension hair found within the ½ cm square section. The top of the resin bond sits at the bottom of the section of natural hair. This section size is used when applying extensions to create a natural-looking, loose free-flowing hairstyle.

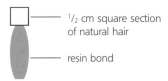

½ cm square section of natural hair

resin bond

A 1 cm square section of natural hair is taken. The same amount of extension hair is drawn to the quantity of extension hair found within the 1 cm square section. The top of the bond sits at the bottom of the section of natural hair. This section size is used when creating loose, free-flowing braids.

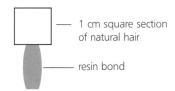

1 cm square section of natural hair

resin bond

A 2 cm square section of natural hair is taken. The same amount of extension hair is drawn to the quantity of extension hair found within the 2 cm square section. The corners of the section are rounded off so the strain is reduced on the natural hair at these points. This section size is used when creating loose, free-flowing dreadlocks.

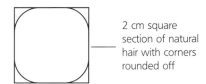

2 cm square section of natural hair with corners rounded off

A ½ cm wide and 2 cm deep rectangle is taken. The same amount of extension hair is drawn to the quantity of extension hair found within the 2 cm square section. The top of the bond sits at the bottom of the section of natural hair. This section size is used when applying extensions to create a natural-looking, loose, free-flowing hairstyle on African-Caribbean hair or other thick and curly natural hair. It condenses the root area to reduce bulk at the scalp.

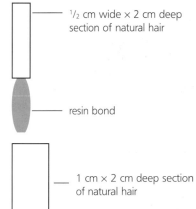

½ cm wide × 2 cm deep section of natural hair

resin bond

A 1 cm wide and 2 cm deep rectangle is taken. The same amount of extension hair is drawn to the quantity of extension hair found within the 2 cm square section. The top of the bond sits at the bottom of the section of natural hair. This section size is used when applying extensions to create a natural-looking, loose, free-flowing hairstyle on African-Caribbean hair or other thick and curly natural hair. It condenses the root area to reduce bulk at the scalp.

1 cm × 2 cm deep section of natural hair

resin bond

A ½ cm wide triangle is taken. The same amount of extension hair is drawn to the quantity of extension hair found within the 2 cm square section. The top of the bond sits at the bottom of the section of natural hair. This section size is used when applying extensions to create a natural-looking, loose, free-flowing hairstyle.

½ cm wide triangular sections of natural hair

A 1 cm wide triangle is taken. The same amount of extension hair is drawn to the quantity of extension hair found within the 2 cm square section. The top of the bond sits at the bottom of the section of natural hair. This section size is used when applying extensions to create a natural-looking, loose, free-flowing hairstyle.

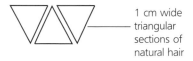

1 cm wide triangular sections of natural hair

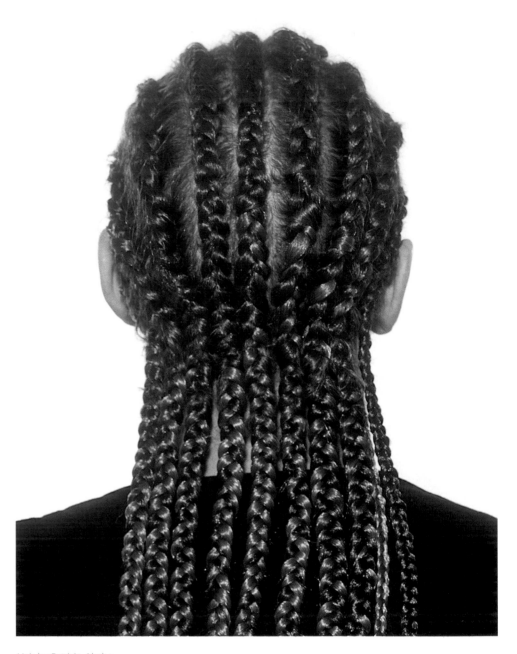

Hair by Patricia Akaba

Cornrows and scalp plaits

Scalp plaits are prepared for the sewing method. An **extension practitioner** can make them as wide or as narrow as desired. Scalp plaits range in width from $\frac{1}{2}$ cm to 2 cm. Scalp plaits contain and condense the natural hair, enabling wefts to be sewn onto it.

When creating natural extension hairstyles you can as much as double the length of the natural hair. If you more than double it, the excessive length will strain the root area where the extension is being held in place. In extreme cases the additional weight can cause the client's natural hair to break during shampooing and brushing, or even to be pulled from the roots.

Always use slightly smaller extensions on top of the client's hair behind the hairline and under the parting, as small extensions are undetectable. The hair is slightly finer at the hairline parting and around the crown so smaller extensions are more suitable.

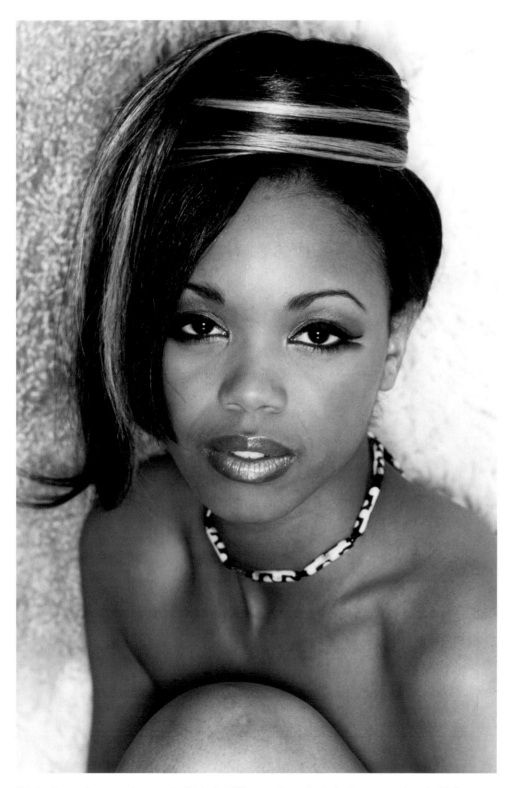

Hair by George Paterson, photography Malcolm Willison, make-up by Suzie Kennett, products by Wella

Knowledge review

1 Why are extensions placed in the interior of natural hair?

2 How far away from a parting should extensions be placed?

3 How many areas are there on the head that extensions can be placed?

4 What is a solid row used for?

5 What does visual placement mean?

6 What is the most used extension size?

7 When would a triangular extension shape be used?

8 What is the ratio of natural hair to extension hair when making a single extension?

9 If a client has 12 cm of natural hair how long can it be extended and why?

10 Why are small extensions used near the hairline and crown?

chapter 8

THE APPLICATION OF HAIR EXTENSIONS

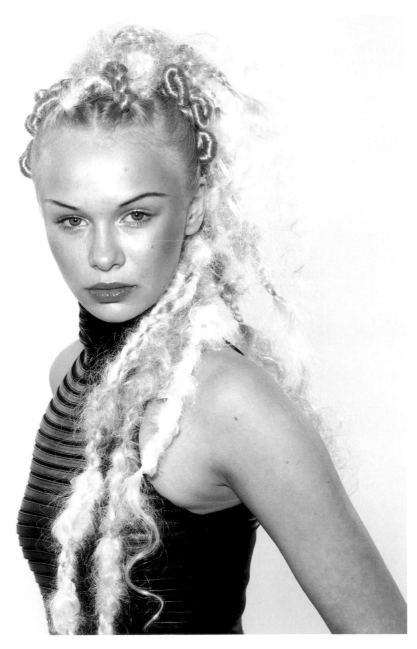

Hair by Theresa Bullock and Jason Smith for aX10 Hair Extension Training

Learning objectives

This chapter covers the application of a variety of hair extension hairstyles, using several extension systems and working on a variety of natural hair types.

- **how to prepare natural hair before applying the extensions**
- **how to prepare extension hair before applying extensions**
- **understand the pre-cutting and post-cutting techniques used for this service**
- **the different application processes for each extension system**
- **the planning and placement of each extension hairstyle**
- **the styling techniques to use on real hair and fibre hair**
- **understand the time each hairstyle takes to apply**
- **see the difference between hair addition, enhancement, extension and alternative hairstyles**

KAORI – HAIR ADDITIONS

Hair additions by Theresa Bullock; extension products by Hair Development Ltd UK.

This extension hairstyle took $1\frac{1}{2}$ hours to complete.

Kaori has virgin hair as her natural hair had no chemical treatments applied. The condition and porosity of the natural hair is normal.

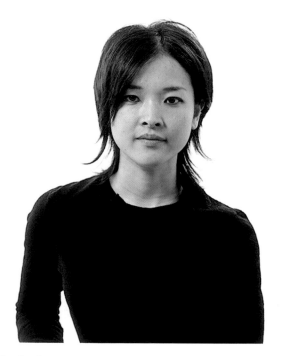

Kaori – before

Preparing the natural hair

Slices of mild bleach are applied into areas 2, 5 and 6 in order to pre-lighten Kaori's hair.

Kaori's natural hair is pre-cut using a **spiral tapering** technique. Spiral tapering takes out blunt lines and ensures that the natural hair will blend with the extension hair. Spiral tapering allows layers in the hair, without removing any of the length. Natural hair is taken in small sections and twisted. Using hairdressing scissors, slice at three points of the twist – the root area, mid-length then the end.

Make very small incisions to ensure that none of the length is removed.

Preparing the extension hair

The hair used to create this enhanced look is Asian extension hair prepared on a machine-sewn weft. Three colours are used: natural black and dark brown that matches the natural hair and bright burgundy used as a block colour. The burgundy will blend with the flashes of colour in the natural hair. The texture of the extension hair used is soft wave as it retains body after blow-drying and the use of straightening irons.

> **REMEMBER** !
>
> Before applying extensions always cleanse with a clarifying shampoo to remove any product residue or oils. Avoid using conditioner and other styling products prior to the extension application!

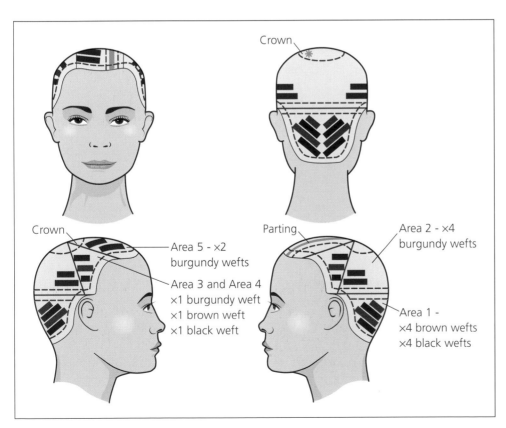

Applying the extension hair

This hairstyle is created using a cold-fusion system, a spirit-based gum called **liquid gold**. The natural hair is parted into the area sections to have extensions applied.

REMEMBER

Always place extensions 2 cm away from the hairline!

Starting in area 1, the wefts applied in this triangle are dark brown and natural black. Alternate the colours in this area to add 2 cm of length to the back of the hairstyle.

TOP TIP

Liquid gold fuses when it dries, but can still be moved around while it is wet. This allows the practitioner more time to place the weft exactly where the hair will fall. Using a hairdryer or heated tongs dry the liquid gold to hold the weft firm.

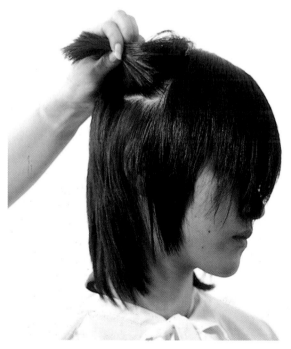

Preparing the natural hair
A vibrant burgundy permanent colour is applied over the pre-lightened slices to match the extension hair colour selected.

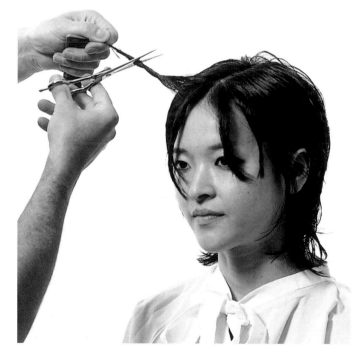

Hair is pre-cut using spiral tapering technique.

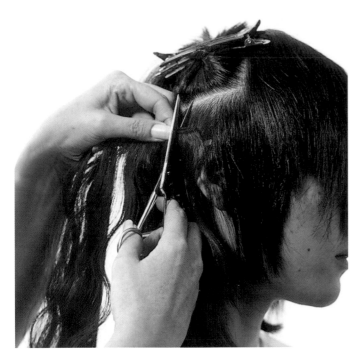

Applying the extension hair
In area two, place the weft next to the section and measure the width then cut the weft to size.

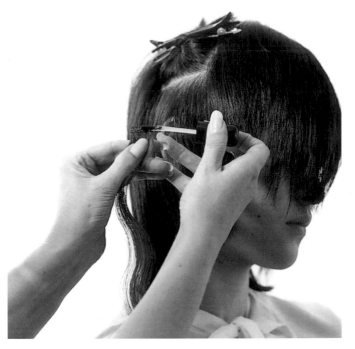

After cutting the weft to size paint the spirit gum onto the thread of the weft at the root area.

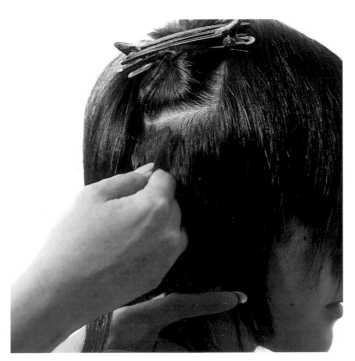

Directionally place the weft on to the natural hair. The natural hair will be carefully placed over the weft so that the join between the extension hair and the natural hair is undetectable.

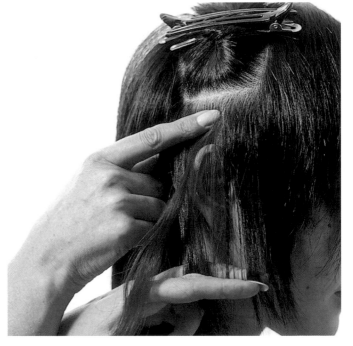

Ensure the weft is placed 1 cm away from the scalp so that it does not come into contact with the skin, and press firmly to secure.

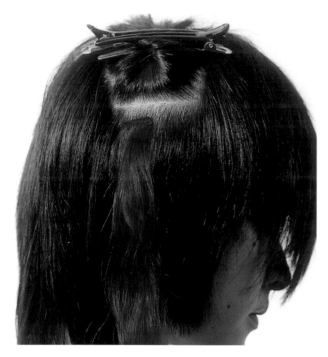

The weft is placed exactly where the hall will fall.

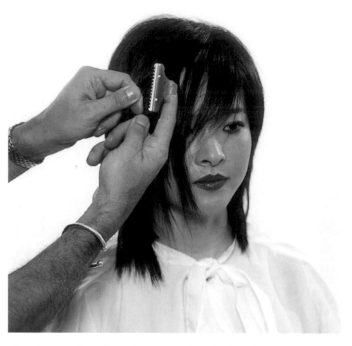

Cutting and styling the extension hairstyle
The hairstyle is blow-dried straight. It is then cut using a **finger razor** and a **flat tapering technique**. See photos of this technique on page 110.

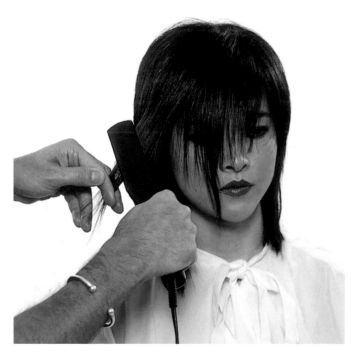

Straightening irons are used to smooth the wavy extension textures and blend the extension hair and natural hair together.

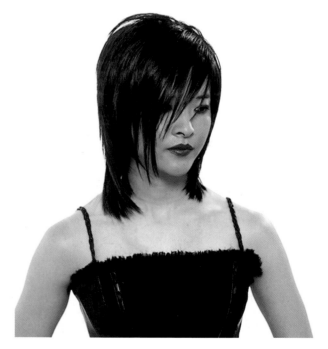

A gel wax is applied to the ends to give definition and shine.

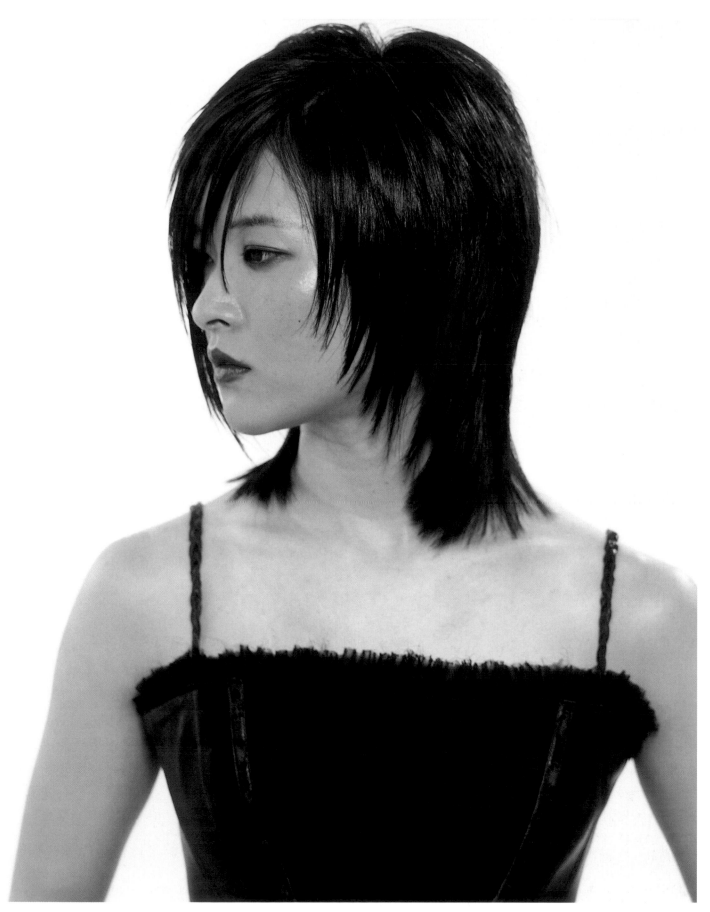

Hair by Theresa Bullock for Hair Development Ltd.

ANGEL – HAIR ADDITIONS

Hair additions by Theresa Bullock, extension products by Mane Connection

Angel's addition hairstyle took 45 minutes to complete.

For this subtle addition hairstyle, straight real European extension hair and a heated dispenser expelling a hot polymer resin is used.

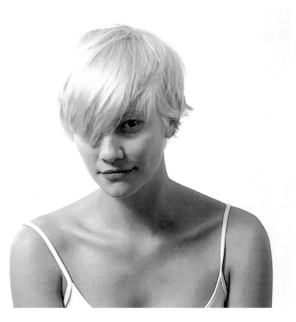

Angel – before

> **REMEMBER** !
>
> Dry natural hair thoroughly before applying extensions, as wet hair will weaken the resin bonds.

Preparing the natural hair

Angel arrived with tinted hair. Using a high lift tint her root regrowth application is completed and slices of an ash tone are applied in area 5.

A small quantity of the real extension hair is coloured using a semi-permanent colour adding a violet ash tone. No pre-cutting is necessary and Angel's hair is dried thoroughly.

Preparing the extension hair

Two extension hair colours: 50 per cent palest blonde, 50 per cent lightest gold blonde and the violet ash tone are placed in a mixing mat.

Applying the extension hair

Extensions are applied in a triangular section in area 5. Five strands are placed in a solid row at the base of the triangle. Working up towards the point of the triangle one less extension strand is applied in each row so that there are 5 at the base, 4 in the row above, 3 in the next row and so on. These rows sit in a **brickwork** fashion to each other, 1 cm apart. The colours are alternated in this area section. Four violet extension strands are placed in area 4.

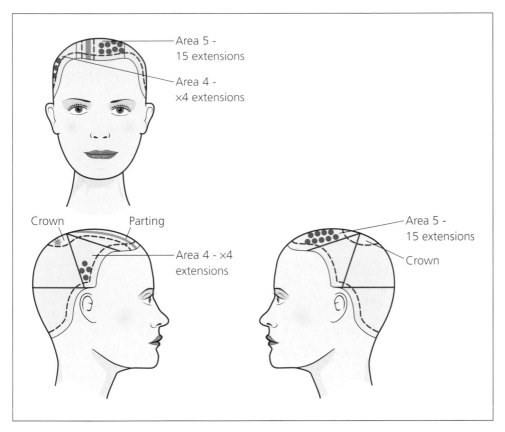

Oxford Designers & Illustrators

Cutting and styling the extension hairstyle

Using tapering scissors, randomly slice the extension hair to remove bulk, ensuring that the extension hair looks as fine as Angel's natural hair. The fringe area is point cut around the perimeter with hairdressing scissors to shape it in asymmetric design. Root-lift is achieved using an **airstyler** to give a subtle bend to the extension hair.

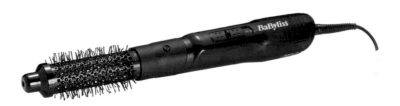

An airstyler Babyliss

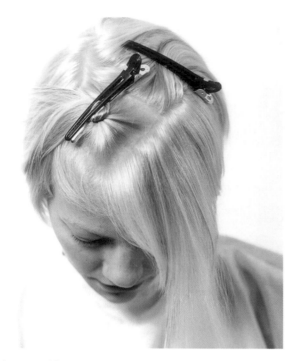

Prepared natural hair

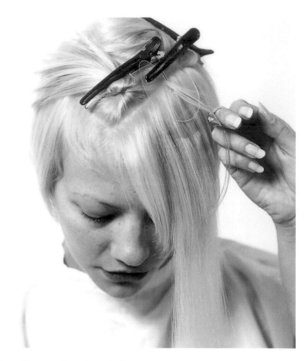

Applying the extension hair
½ cm-square sections of natural hair are taken in each row with a scalp shield secured over these sections.

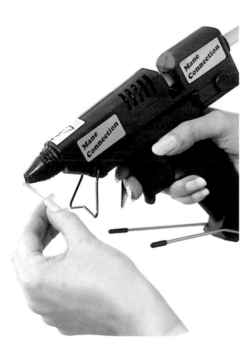

Drawing equal quantities of extension hair and natural hair, dispense a drop of hot resin on the root area of the extension hair.

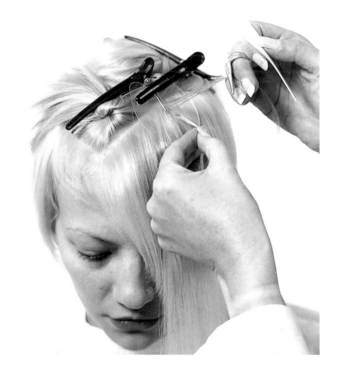

Prepared extension hair, ready to place.

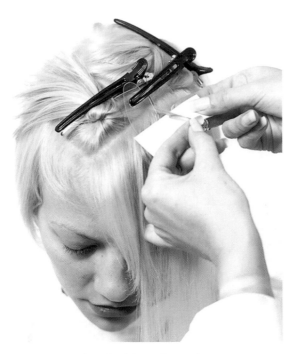

Taking the extension that holds resin at the root area to the natural hair and using a silicone pad, press the resin through the natural hair.

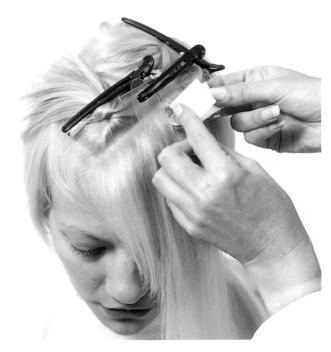

Fold the silicone pad in half. A bond is rolled the size and shape of a grain of rice, sealing and securing the extension strand in place $\frac{1}{2}$ cm away from the scalp at the root area of the natural hair.

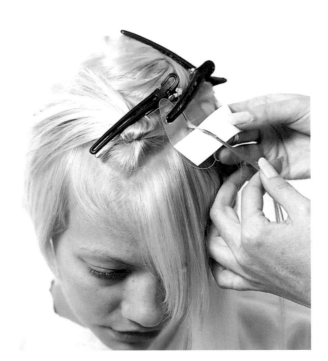

Extension hair has bonded to the natural hair.

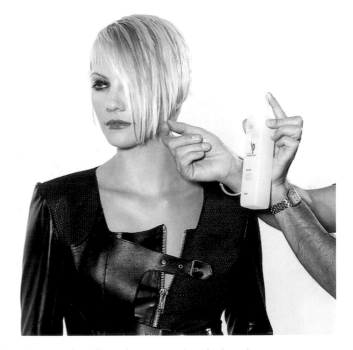

Cutting and styling the extension hairstyle
A light fixing spray is applied and a small amount of gel wax is used on the tips to control the fine hair. This application gives the model a fringe 3 cm longer than her natural hair and violet hi-lights.

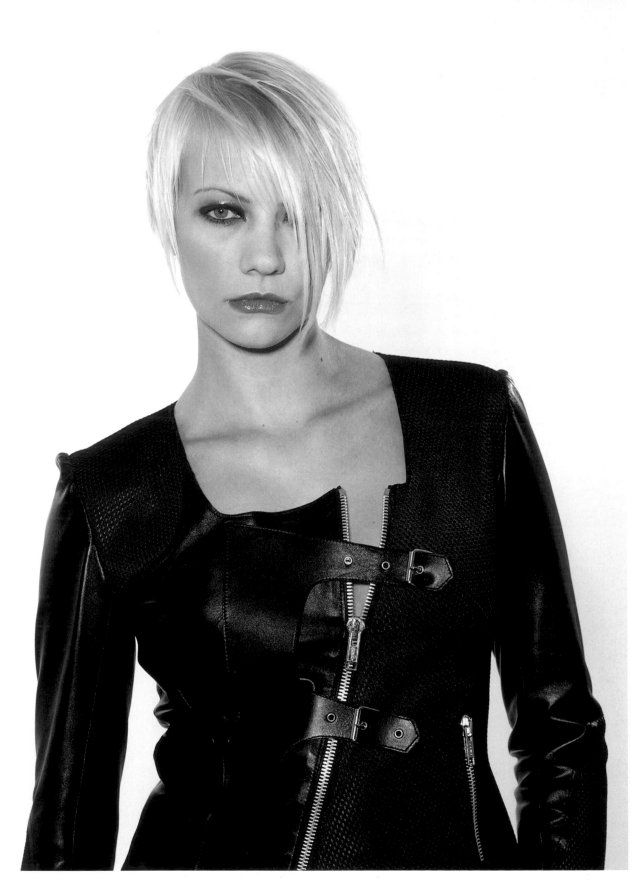

Hair by Theresa Bullock for Mane Connection

FAY – HAIR ENHANCEMENT

Hair enhancements by Ann Fegan for H²D4, extension products by Racoon International

This hairstyle took 2 hours to complete.

This distinctive enhancement hairstyle was created using Racoon's hot-bond system and real European extension hair.

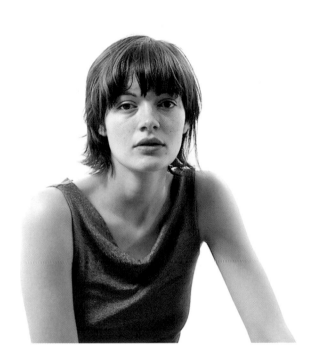

Fay – before

Preparing the natural hair

Fay's natural hair is coloured using a semi-permanent warm tone colour. It is then blow-dried.

Preparing the extension hair

Three extension hair colours are used: dark brown, warm brown and deep copper to match Fay's natural hair; 60 per cent of dark brown extension hair is used with 20 per cent each of the warm colours to create the desired colour. The extension hair is kept cuticle correct before application. The real extension hair is attached as individual strands to ensure a free-flowing, authentic-looking hairstyle.

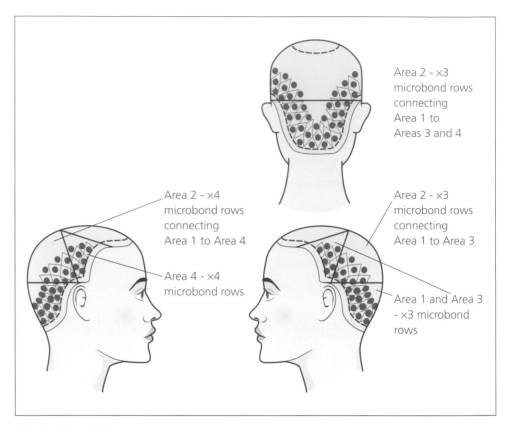

Oxford Designers & Illustrators

Area 2 - ×3 microbond rows connecting Area 1 to Areas 3 and 4

Area 2 - ×4 microbond rows connecting Area 1 to Area 4

Area 4 - ×4 microbond rows

Area 2 - ×3 microbond rows connecting Area 1 to Area 3

Area 1 and Area 3 - ×3 microbond rows

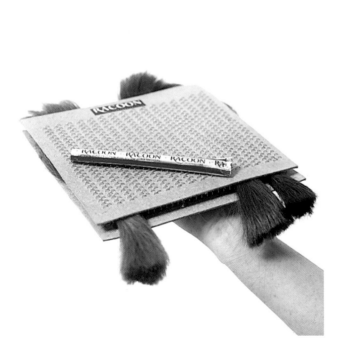

Preparing the extension hair
The three extension hair colours are placed in the mixing mat to mix them into one strand.

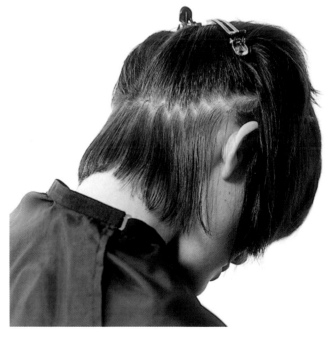

Applying the extension hair
The extension hair is directionally placed 1–2 cm away from the hairline in triangular sections. Extensions are directionally placed in areas 1, 3 and 4 placing individual strands to fall forward.

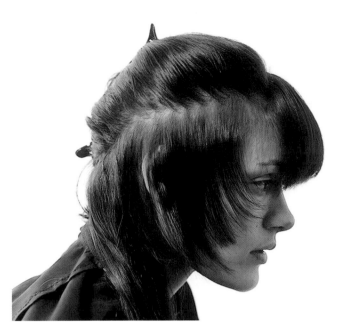

Extensions are applied at the top and bottom of the longest point of the triangle. This is called **microbonding**.

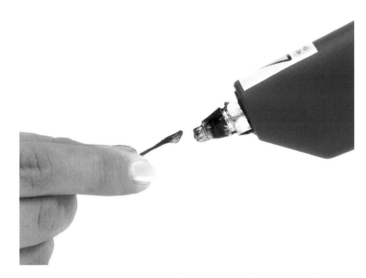

Taking an equal amount of extension hair, use a hot melt dispenser that dispenses hot resin onto the root end of the extension hair.

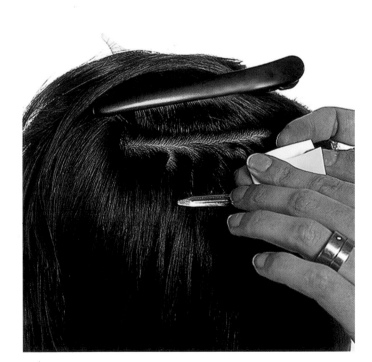

Attach the extension hair to the real hair.

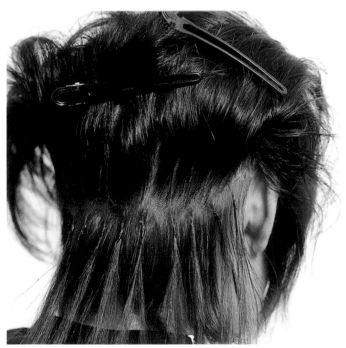

Extensions are placed 1 cm away from the scalp at the root area of the natural hair, creating a resin bond. A silicone pad is used to roll and seal the bond.

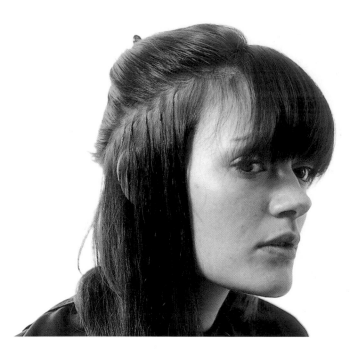

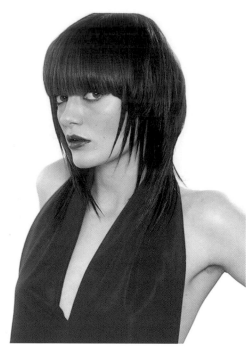

Three microbond rows are applied in area 3 and four rows in area 4. By adding more extension hair in area 4, an asymmetrical style is achieved.

The extension hair is cut using a razor, to give the hairstyle a layered, jagged look and the model's fringe is blunt cut to frame her face. Using straightening irons connects the hair textures..

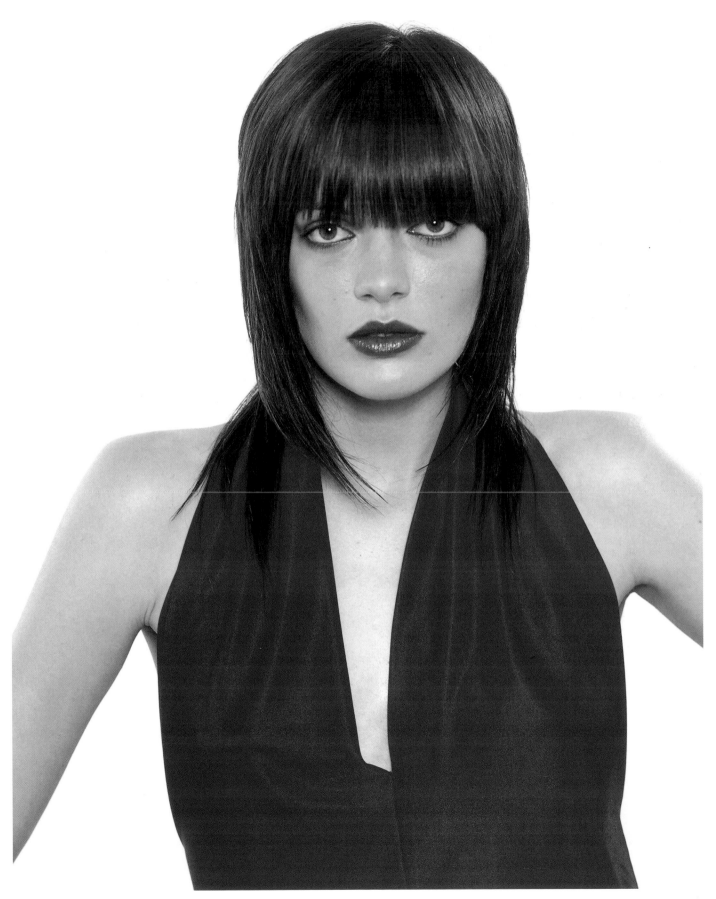

Hair by Anne Fegan at H²D4 for Racoon International

LAURA – HAIR ENHANCEMENT

Hair enhancements by Jason Smith, extension products by Eurohair Fashion UK, Pierre Balmain Extensions

This hairstyle took 2 hours to complete.

Body and volume are achieved in this hairstyle using real extension hair strips, wefts and a hot-bond system – **heat sealing**. Laura has highlights in her natural hair; it is fine and in need of thickness.

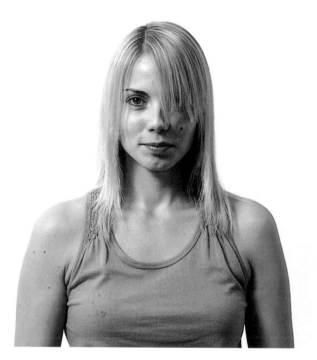

Laura – before

Preparing the extension hair

Real extension hair is used on a hand-sewn **hair strip** (small weft). No mixing is required as a blonde colour is used to match the natural hair colour.

Applying the extension hair

Section the natural hair, taking the front sections out of the way first. Use four hair strips to create this look, placing the first in area 1, just under the occipital bone and one on either side of the model's head, in areas 3 and 4. Half a strip is placed either side of Laura's head in areas 5 and 6.

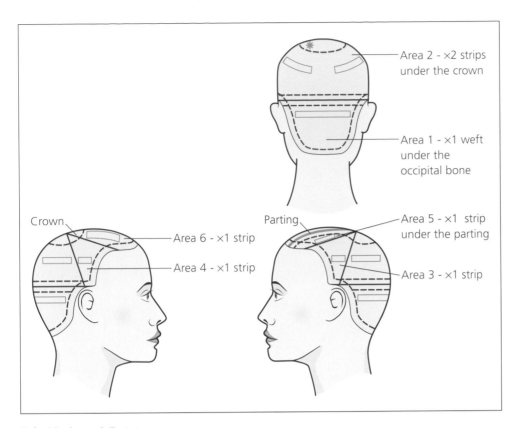

Area 2 - ×2 strips under the crown

Area 1 - ×1 weft under the occipital bone

Crown

Area 6 - ×1 strip

Area 4 - ×1 strip

Parting

Area 5 - ×1 strip under the parting

Area 3 - ×1 strip

Oxford Designers & Illustrators

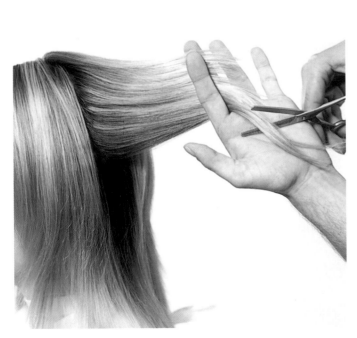

Preparing the natural hair
Thinning scissors are used to taper the ends of the natural hair and remove any hard lines.

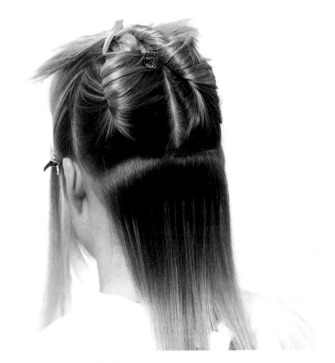

Section the natural hair.

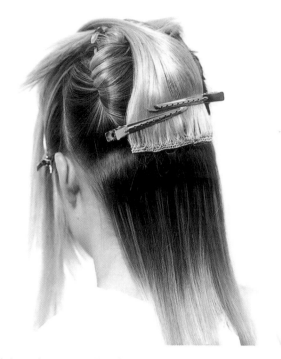

Applying the extension hair
The strip is placed up to the natural hair and pinned upside-down.

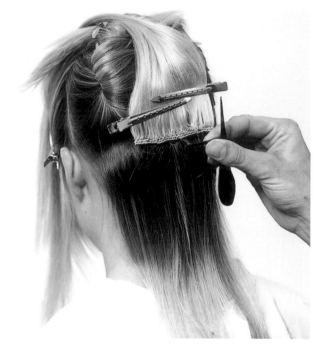

Highlights of natural hair are pulled through five holes in the hair strip using a crochet hook.

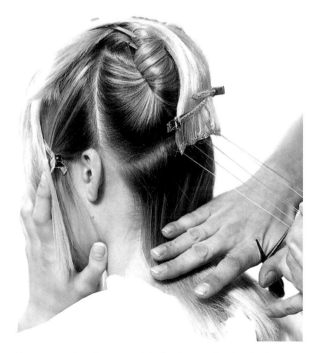

Pulling the strands of natural hair through the hair strip.

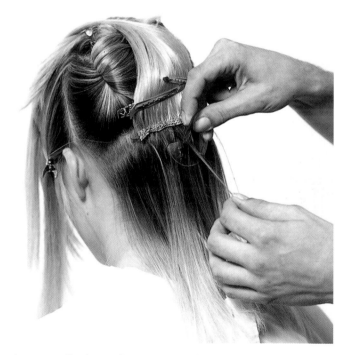

Take a small triangular section of natural hair directly underneath the pulled through strand and hold the two strands together.

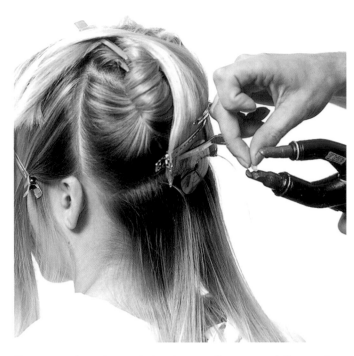

Put some bond wax into the applicator and then wipe the wax onto the two pieces of natural hair.

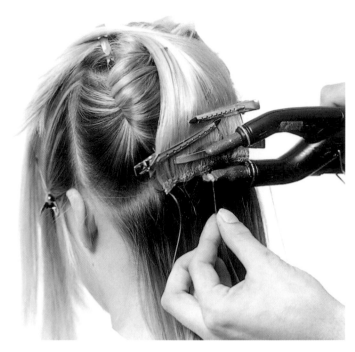

Applying the extension hair to the natural hair using a hot-bond applicator.

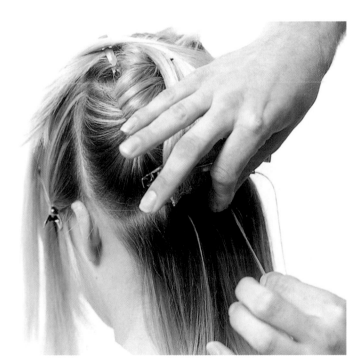

Using thumb and index finger to roll the wax, make sure that the top and bottom of the wax are closed so that the bond looks like a grain of rice. When rolling the wax, the practitioner's fingernails should be pointing to the floor so that the wax comes away from the head and to ensure that the bond is not too tight. Polish the bond with the connector to check that the bond is sealed. This gives the attachment a cleaner finish.

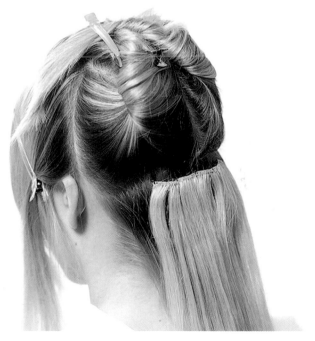

This same process is repeated for all five strands. Unpin the hair strip so that it falls down (**root point perfect**) and covers all of the bonds for a natural effect.

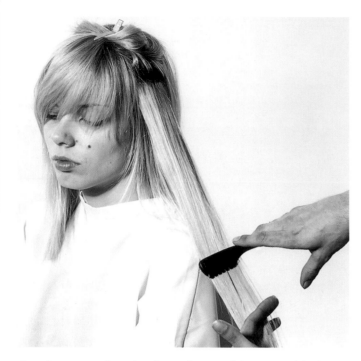

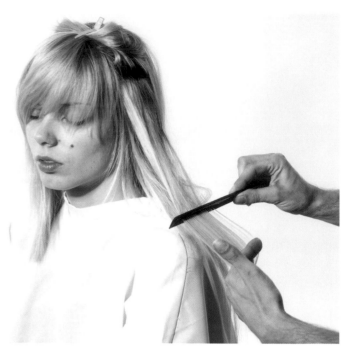

Cut the extensions back to the model's natural hair length. Push the natural hair away and cut the extension hair with a razor using a flat tapering technique.

After cutting, the hair is then blow-dried at the crown to give extra volume and flicked out at the sides and the fringe using a hairdryer and round brush.

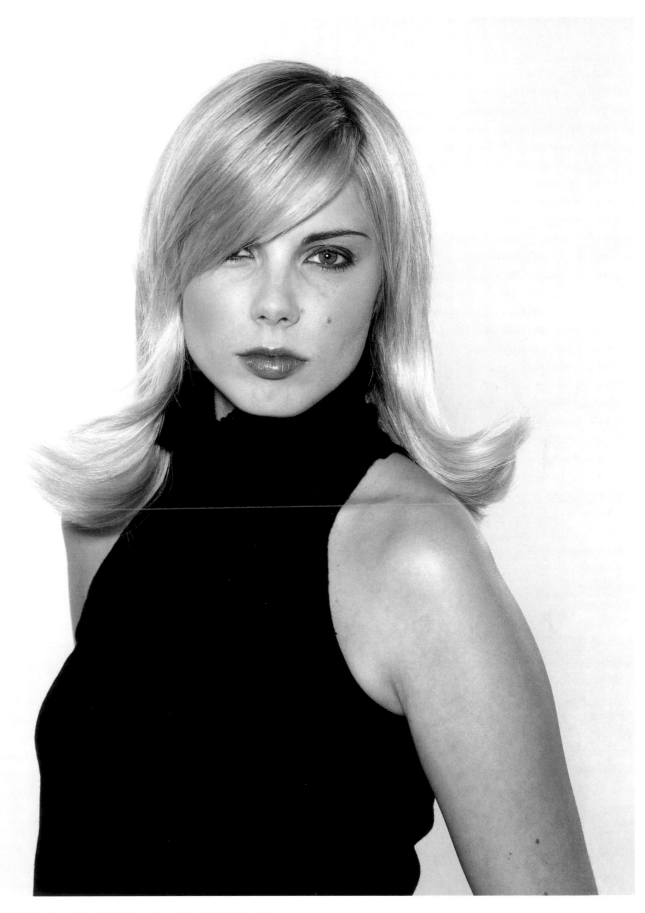

Hair by Jason Smith for Piere Balmain Hair Extensions, Euro Hair Fashion UK

MIA – HAIR EXTENSIONS

Hair extensions by Theresa Bullock for aX10 Hair Extension Training

This style took $2^1/_2$ hours to complete.

This stunning hair extension hairstyle was created using a cold-fusion system with adhesive **tapes** that create a weft and straight fibre extension hair. Mia has virgin hair; extensions are applied into all areas in order to create a lengthened hairstyle. A semi-permanent colour is used in Mia's natural hair to give it shine and to ensure that it matches the fibre extension hair colour.

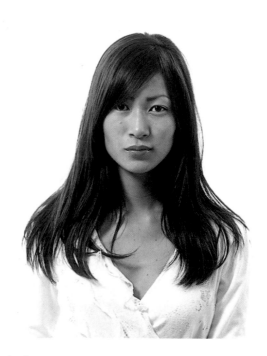

Mia – before

Preparing the extension hair

Three colours are used to create a colour match to the natural hair colour: dark brown, natural black and a dark burgundy; 50 per cent dark brown and 25 per cent each of natural black and dark burgundy fibre were brushed and blended together. Spray the fibre with a de-tangling spray and brush it thoroughly, blending all three colours together. This is called mega-mixing.

A titian fibre colour is added to the hairstyle as a contrast to give highlights. The fibre is then made into a weft using adhesive tape.

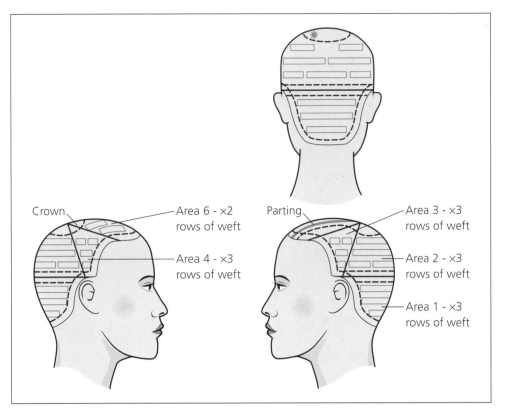

Crown
Area 6 - ×2 rows of weft
Parting
Area 3 - ×3 rows of weft
Area 4 - ×3 rows of weft
Area 2 - ×3 rows of weft
Area 1 - ×3 rows of weft

Oxford Designers & Illustrators

Cutting and styling the extension hairstyle

REMEMBER !

Straight or blunt cuts will make fibre look false, as it does not behave in the same way as natural hair.

After the extensions have been applied, the ends of the fibre are trimmed. The fibre is point cut around the perimeter using hairdressing scissors to create a natural **baseline**. Some of the weight of the hairstyle is removed using a razor. Finally, the hairstyle is dressed using gel to add definition.

TOP TIP

Never use your best pair of hairdressing scissors to cut fibre extension hair, as it will damage them.

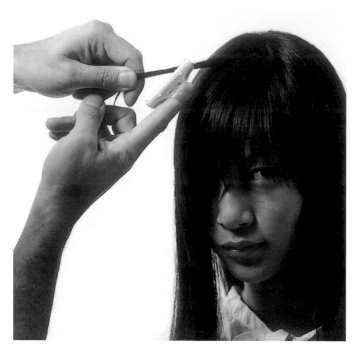

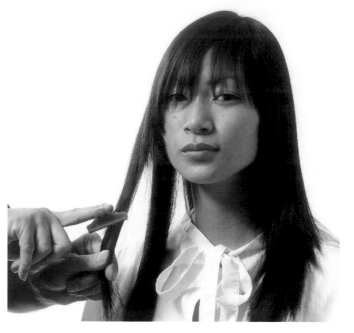

Preparing the natural hair
Taper the hair using thinning scissors to soften the edges and use a finger razor to flat taper the fringe area and remove any straight blunt cut lines so that the fibre will blend with the natural hair.

Preparing the natural hair.

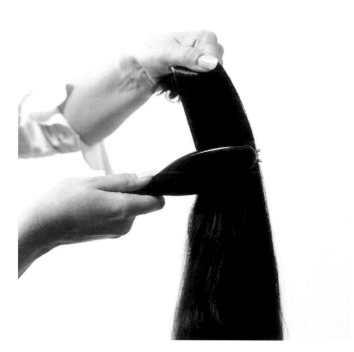

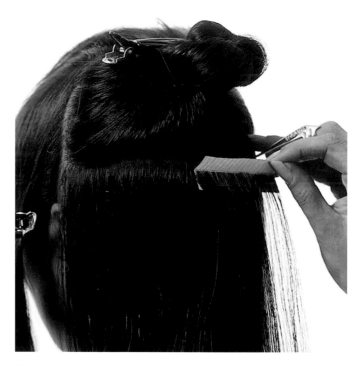

Mega-mixing the extension hair colours together.

The wefts are applied. The practitioner uses a **Mclau** on her finger to help take straight clean sections of hair. The weft is measured to the same width as the hair section and cut to size using an old pair of hairdressing scissors.

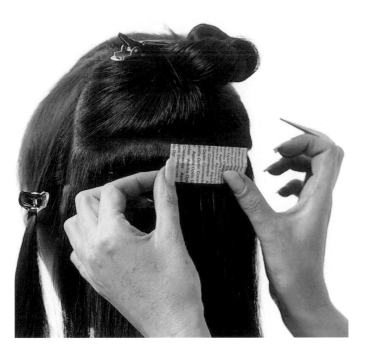

Apply the weft directly onto the natural hair.

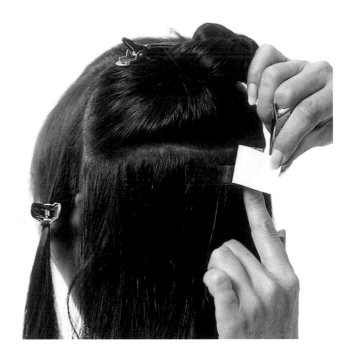

Applying the extension hair.

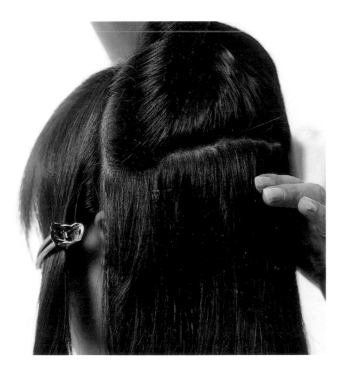

Take a fine section of natural hair (about ¼ cm) above the tape and drop it down over the tape, pressing the natural hair to the topside of the tape to ensure that the weft is secure and that the tape is undetectable. Follow the same procedure in areas 2, 3 and 4, before placing the titian highlights into areas 5 and 6.

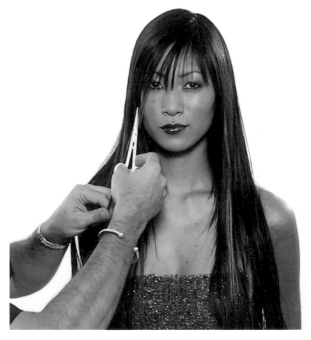

The titian fibre is applied by cutting 1 cm square sections of the tape and placing it visually.

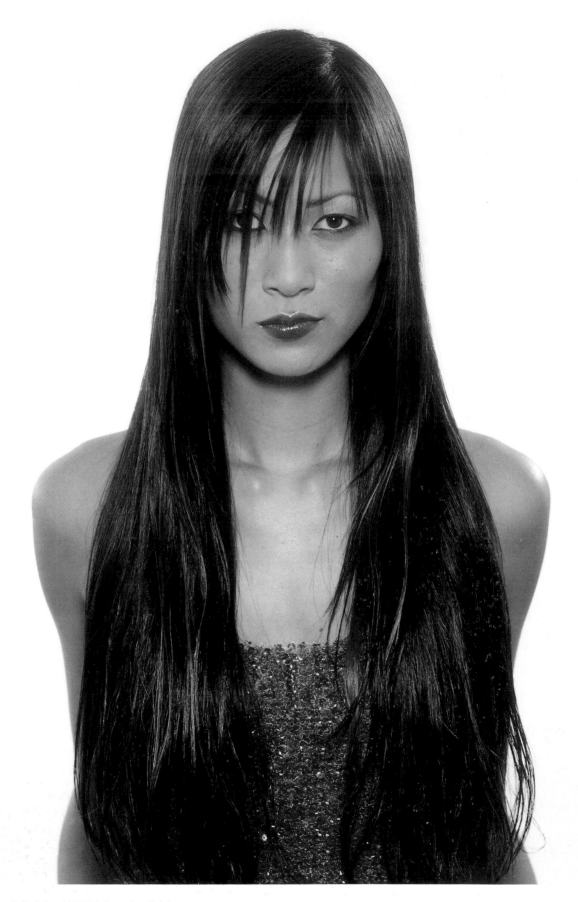

Hair by Theresa Bullock for aX10 Hair Extension Training

KAMILLA – HAIR EXTENSIONS

Hair extensions by Marie Marcel, extension products by Cinderella Hair

This hairstyle took four hours to complete.

To achieve this truly fairytale look, pre-bonded real European extension hair strands and a hot-bond system are used. With this system, the practitioner rolls the adhesive bond using the thumb and forefinger as the bond is not hot.

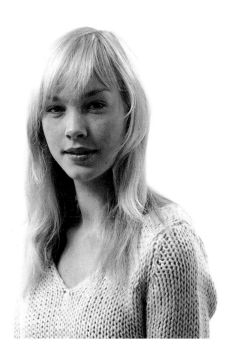

Kamilla – before

Preparing the natural hair

Kamilla's hair is highlighted using a high lift tint and is then trimmed using thinning scissors at the ends to reduce blunt lines. It is rough-dried to give a natural look retaining a wavy texture.

Preparing the extension hair

Two colours to match the natural hair are selected: ash blonde and light blonde. These colours are pre-blended.

> **REMEMBER** !
>
> This service can not be learnt from a video or books alone. Always attend professional training courses to learn the practical skills required.

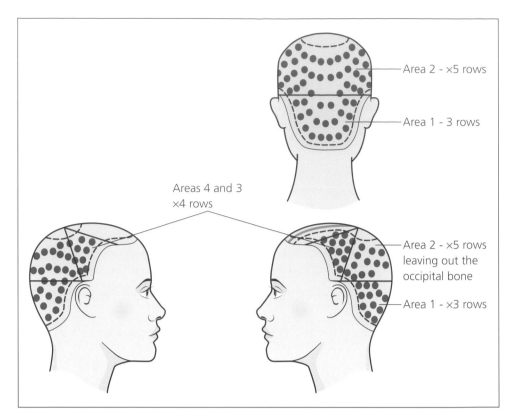

Area 2 - ×5 rows

Area 1 - 3 rows

Areas 4 and 3
×4 rows

Area 2 - ×5 rows
leaving out the
occipital bone

Area 1 - ×3 rows

Oxford Designers & Illustrators

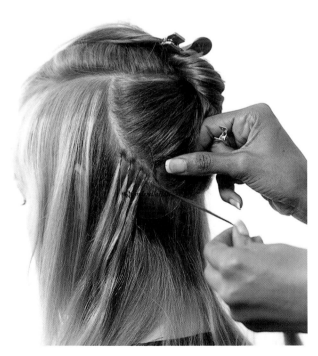

The natural hair is sectioned and the extensions are applied onto 1 cm square sections of natural hair. A scalp shield is attached to the natural hair to protect it from the heated applicator.

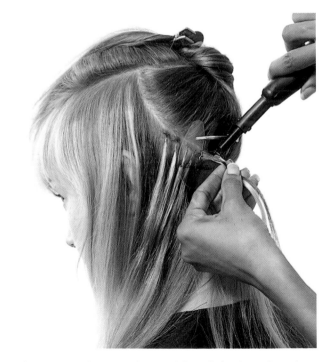

Place the natural hair in the middle of the bond and seal it using a heated applicator.

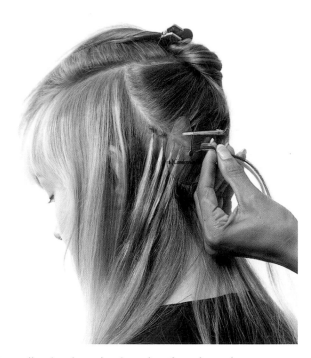

Roll the adhesive bond using the thumb and forefinger

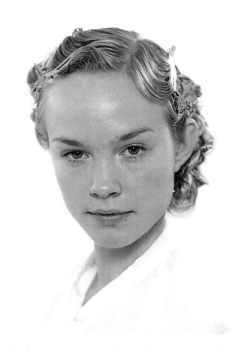

Once all of the extensions have been applied, the hair is pinned up using a combination of finger waves, pin curls and barrel curls.

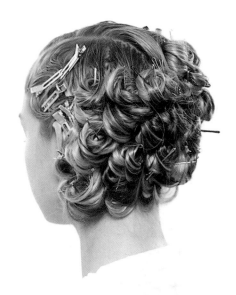

The practitioner uses pin curl clips for the pin curls and kirby grips to secure the barrel curls.

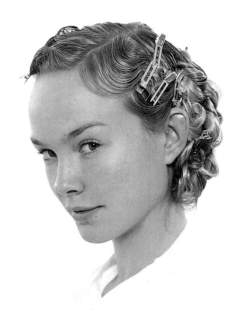

These very traditional setting techniques are then fixed with hairspray. The style is set under a hood dryer for twenty minutes. The clips are then removed to reveal a very feminine, tousled look.

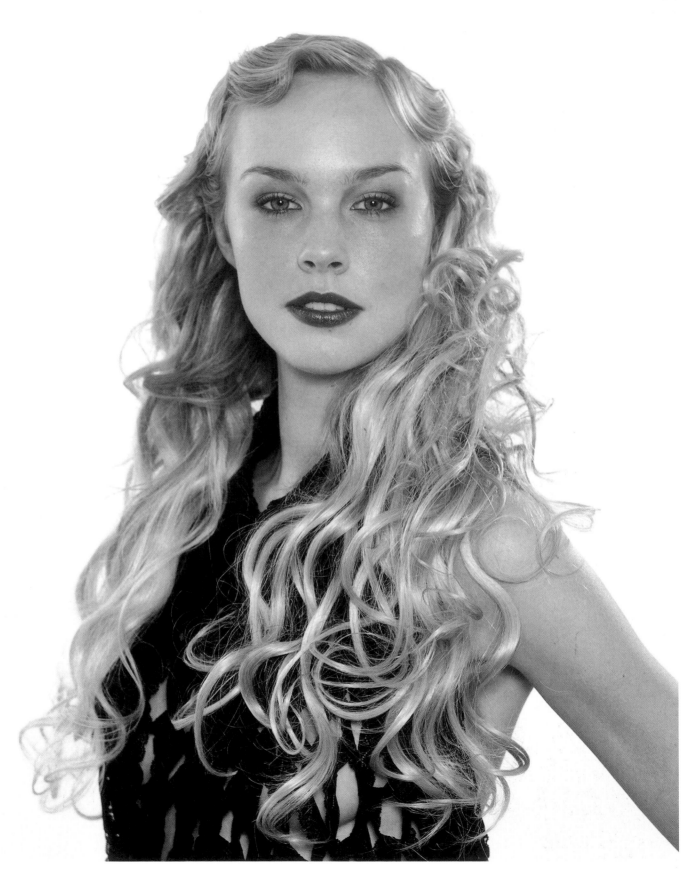

Hair by Marie Marcel for Cinderella Hair

NINA – HAIR EXTENSIONS

Hair extensions by Marie Marcel for aX10 Hair Extension Training

This style took 2¹/₂ hours to complete.

Nina's natural hair is relaxed with a 2 cm **root** regrowth of virgin hair.

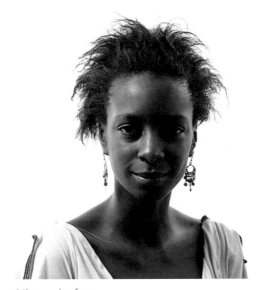

Nina – before

Preparing the natural hair

Nina's hair is blow-dried as straight as possible. This is achieved using a small-tooth Afro-comb and some beeswax. Gel helps to keep the hair flat at the hairline.

Preparing the extension hair

The hair used is 50 per cent dark brown extension hair by Cinderella hair and 50 per cent highlighted blonde and dark brown extension hair. This straight extension hair is on a fine hand-sewn weft.

> **REMEMBER** !
>
> To ensure that the extension hair will blend with the natural hair, use thinning scissors to thin or taper the ends of the natural hair and remove any hard lines before applying extensions.

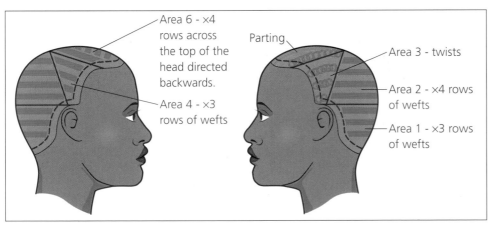

Area 6 - ×4 rows across the top of the head directed backwards.

Area 4 - ×3 rows of wefts

Parting

Area 3 - twists

Area 2 - ×4 rows of wefts

Area 1 - ×3 rows of wefts

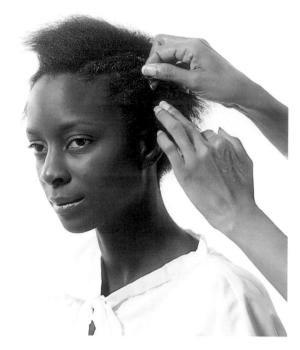

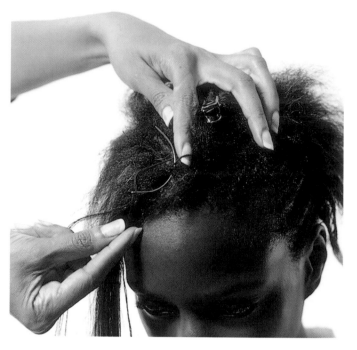

Twists are created in area 3 to draw Nina's hair away from her face. The twists are secured with a clear elastic at the ends and then fixed with a hold-in spray. A straightening iron and wax is used on the remaining natural hair to straighten it, ensuring that the extensions will blend.

Using a curved needle and a silk thread that matches the natural hair colour, sew 1 cm square sections of natural hair then carry the thread to the neighbouring 1 cm square section. This creates a track in a row across the hair.

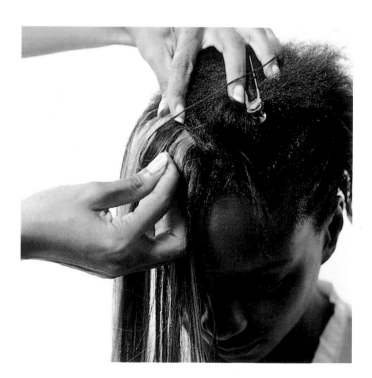

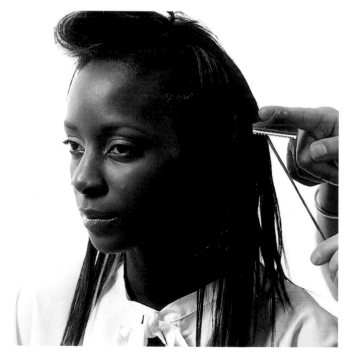

Sew the wefts onto the track of thread.

The hair is cut using a razor to give it a fine look and then finger dressed with hairspray.

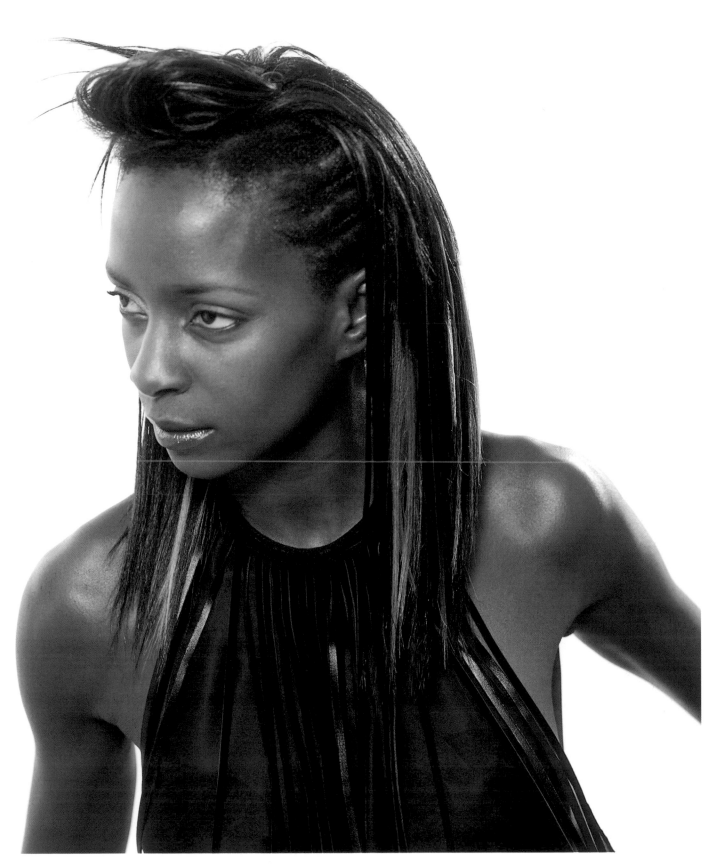

Hair by Marie Marcel for aX10 Hair Extension Training

JONATHON – HAIR ALTERNATIVE

Hair by Patricia Akaba, extension products from American Dream

This hairstyle took 1½ hours to complete.

Patricia created this strong masculine alternative look using a **three-stem braid** and jumbo fibre extension hair.

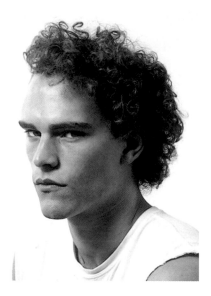

Jonathon – before

Preparing the natural hair

Jonathon's hair is shampooed with a clarifying shampoo to remove any residue, oil, wax and styling products and then blast-dried.

Preparing the extension hair

Two colours of jumbo fibre are used: a mid-copper and a dark brown. Blending extension hair colours is not required for this hairstyle.

Applying the extension hair

This is the only hairstyle in this collection where the stylist starts from the front. A fine piece of fibre is incorporated into the front and at the beginning of the braid.

The braids are applied throughout the model's head. Caucasian hair is very slippery when it is dry so during the braiding process lightly spray water on the natural hair to control and grip the curls. The ends of the braids are sealed using a heat clamp directly on the fibre, which melts it, creating a hard plastic bond. This bond prevents the three-stem braid from unravelling.

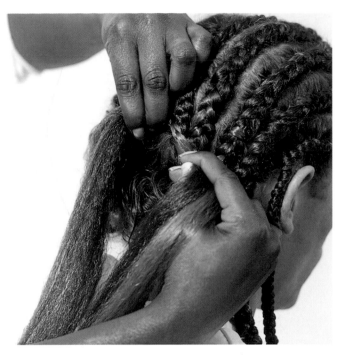

As the braid is created more jumbo fibre is added to thicken it.

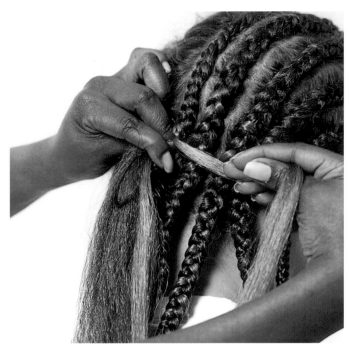

As a decorative feature add the mid-copper fibre to the braid at the nape area.

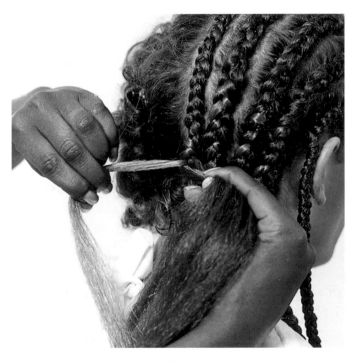

Continue to braid adding fibre to extend Jonathon's hair by 12 cm.

Cutting and styling

Use hairdressing scissors to trim any stray pieces of fibre in the braids.

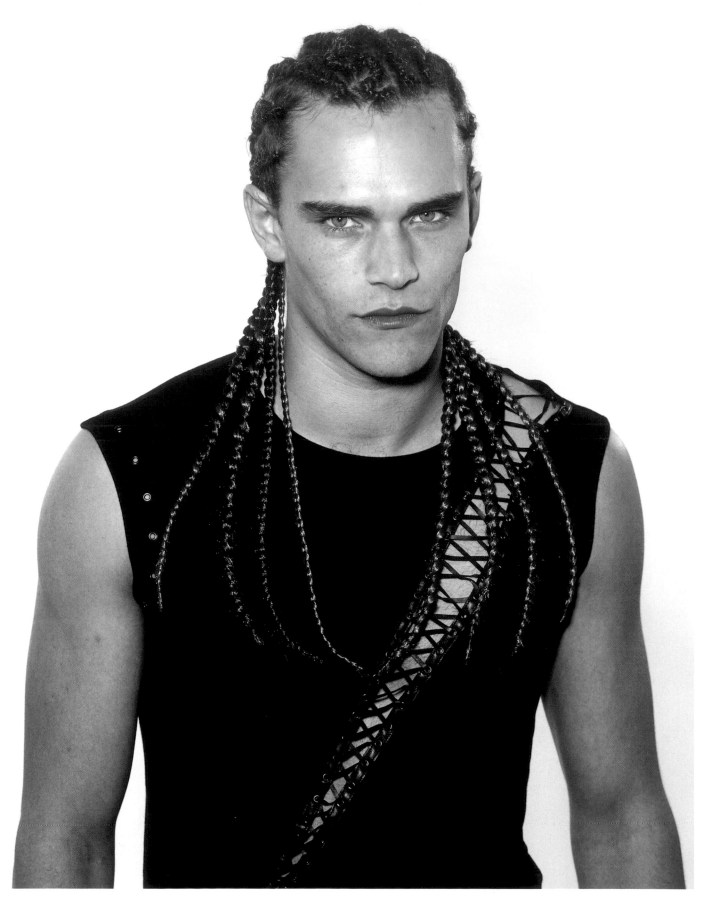

Hair by Patricia Akaba for American Dream

YULIA – HAIR ALTERNATIVE

Hair by Theresa Bullock and Jason Smith, sponsored by aX10 Hair Extension Training

To create this radical alternative look, the stylists used different coloured fibre hair creating **textured** braids. The braids are called **smooth dreadlocks** and backcombed **four-stem braids**.

Two practitioners work together to create the smooth dreadlocks and four-stem braids. These techniques require two stylists, an operator and an assistant.

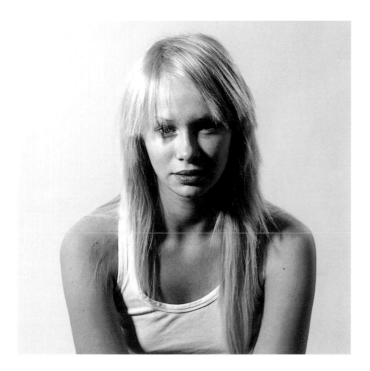

Yulia – before

Preparing the natural hair

Yulia has virgin hair and after cleansing it is rough-dried.

Preparing the extension hair

Three fibre colours are used: cool blonde, pale blonde and strawberry blonde. Three-quarters of the fibre is backcombed in large strands to create the desired texture for the backcombed braids. The remaining fibre is blended into a mega-mix for the smooth dreadlocks.

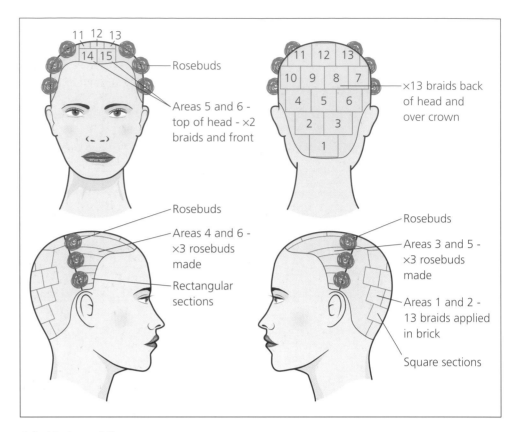

11 12 13
14 15
Rosebuds

Areas 5 and 6 - top of head - ×2 braids and front

11 12 13
10 9 8 7
4 5 6
2 3
1

×13 braids back of head and over crown

Rosebuds

Areas 4 and 6 - ×3 rosebuds made

Rectangular sections

Rosebuds

Areas 3 and 5 - ×3 rosebuds made

Areas 1 and 2 - 13 braids applied in brick

Square sections

Oxford Designers & Illustrators

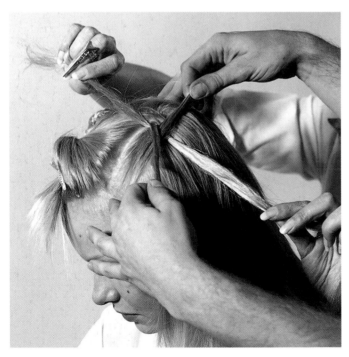

The operator works with the natural hair, taking a large rectangular section and dividing it in two. The assistant works with the smooth fibre applying it into the divide of this section.

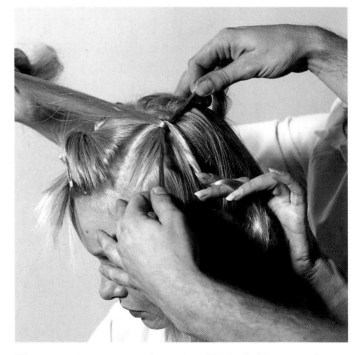

The operator crosses the natural hair right over left and the assistant crosses the fibre left over right.

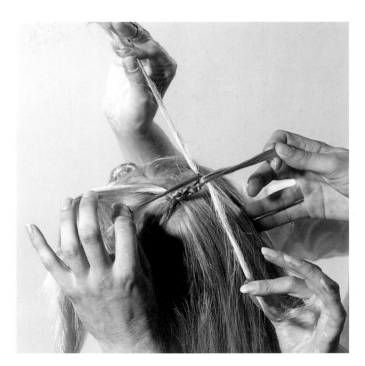

The natural hair is crossed right over left one more time and one piece of fibre is placed over the top of the head and left out of the braid. The remaining piece of fibre that the assistant holds is divided in half and taken through the centre of the braid.

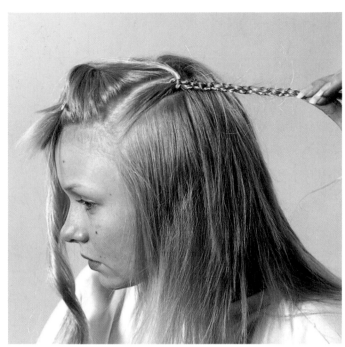

The natural hair is now crossed right over left and the fibre left over right then repeated several times. This creates a four-stem locking braid, which will not unravel.

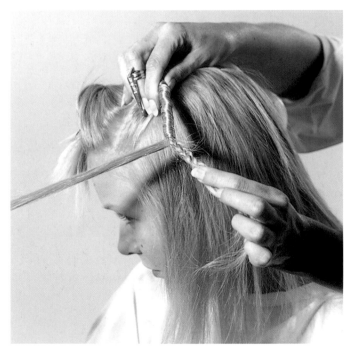

When the braid is 12 cm long, the assistant holds the end of the braid and the operator takes the remaining piece of fibre and wraps it around the held braid.

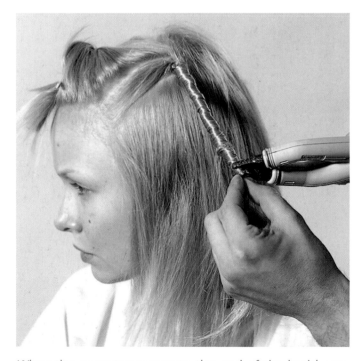

When the operator comes to the end of the braid, use a heat clamp to melt the fibre creating a hard bond, securing the dreadlock at the end (unlike the other processes that are secured at the root). This creates a smooth dreadlock.

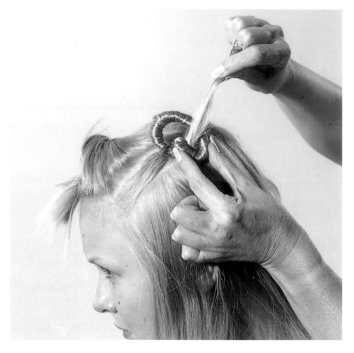

The assistant takes the smooth dreadlock tying it close to the scalp to form a knot that looks like a rosebud.

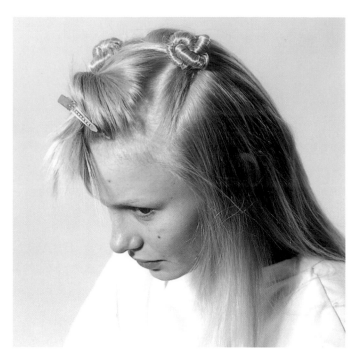

Completed rosebud knot.

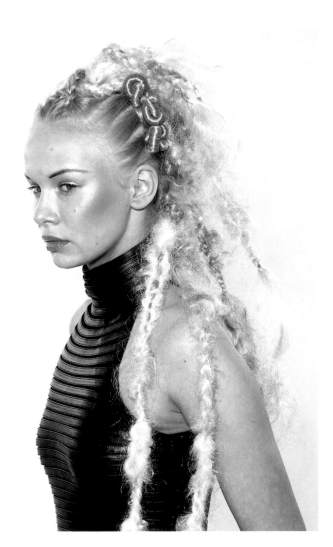

The knots can be used for strong avant-garde looks or bridal hairstyles.

The second technique used on this model is called a backcombed four-stem braid. Backcombed fibre is braided into the natural hair. The operator takes a large section of natural hair and divides it in two. The assistant places the backcombed fibre through the centre. The operator crosses the natural hair right over left, the assistant crosses the backcombed fibre left over right until the braid is as long as required. Additional backcombed fibre is added to lengthen the braid using alternate colours. A heat clamp is used to secure the end of the braid creating a hard bond.

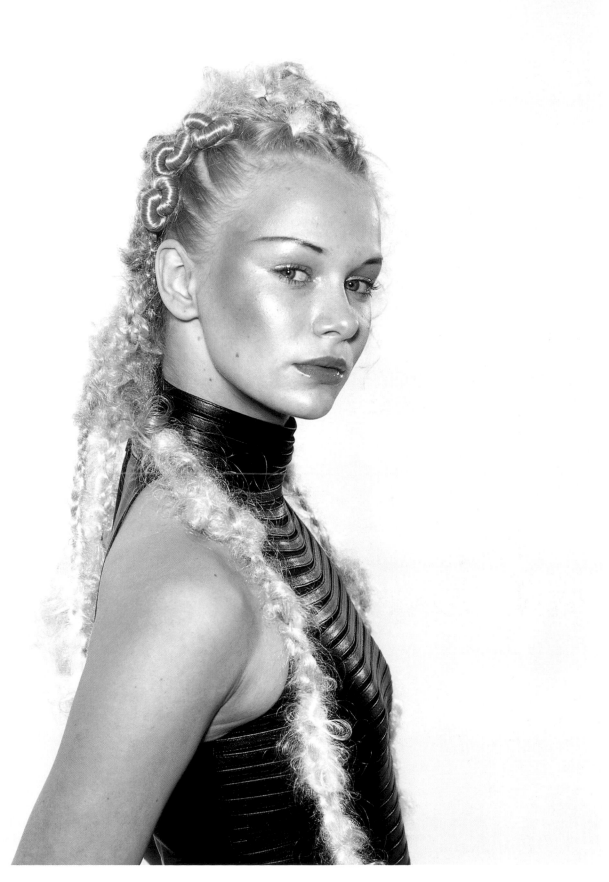

Hair by Theresa Bullock and Jason Smith for aX10 Hair Extension Training

Knowledge review

1 What is spiral tapering?

2 Why are extensions applied $^1/_2$–1 cm away from the scalp when working on Asian, Caucasian and Oriental hair types?

3 What is flat tapering?

4 What heated electrical styling tools can be used on real and fibre hair?

5 What will happen to a hairstyle if extensions are applied on top of the occipital bone?

6 Why is all chemical work conducted before extensions are applied?

7 How is an asymmetric extension hairstyle created?

8 What is the difference between hair additions and hair enhancements?

9 What is the difference between hair extensions and hair alternatives?

10 List the pre-cutting and post-cutting techniques used on the models throughout this chapter.

chapter 9

CLIENT AFTERCARE AND HOMECARE PROCEDURES

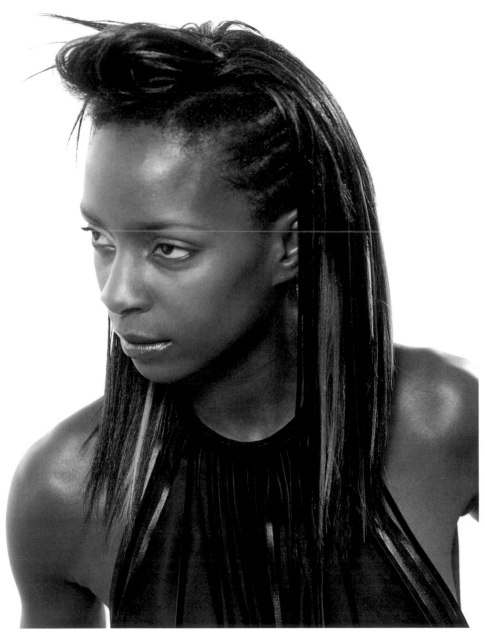

Hair by Marie Marcel for aX10 Hair Extension Training

133

Learning objectives

- **learn how to prepare a client aftercare sheet**
- **homecare procedures for real and fibre hair**
- **introduction to styling procedures for extension hair**
- **how to advise clients about homecare procedures**

CLIENT AFTERCARE PROCEDURES

Before offering the hair extension service, prepare client aftercare sheets. These are worksheets to give to a client containing homecare advice and maintenance tips. These are **aftercare requirements**.

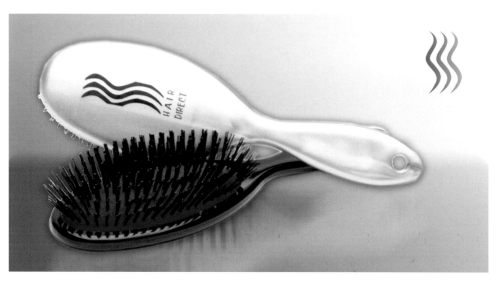

Hair Direct

CLIENT AFTERCARE PROCEDURES

- Shampoo the hair extension hairstyle no less than 24 hours after application.
- Before shampooing the hair extension hairstyle brush the hair with the soft bristle brush.
- Begin brushing the ends of the hairstyle in downward strokes, moving up the hair until finally placing the brush at the root area and brushing thoroughly and firmly from the root through to the ends.
- Before shampooing **separate the bonds**, one from the other, at the root area. The extension bonds can stick together or hair at the root area can entwine between the bonds and lock together.
- Shampoo at least twice a week. This is to ensure that natural oils do not build up at the scalp area. This natural oil is called sebum. Sebum is an acid solution, sitting on the pH scale between 4.5 and 5.5 and can break down some of the polymer resins or bond adhesives attaching the extensions in place.

CLIENT AFTERCARE PROCEDURES continued

- Use the cleansing and conditioning products recommended specifically for the extension system applied. Speak to the practitioner for aftercare product advice.
- Standing in a shower is an ideal position for shampooing an extension hairstyle as the water and the hair flow in a vertical downward direction.
- Wet the natural hair and extension hair together. Apply the clarifying shampoo throughout the hairstyle. Using fingertips massage the shampoo gently at the scalp area and stroke the shampoo into the extension hair to the tips. Rinse the hair thoroughly using clean running water and gently squeeze the extension hairstyle to remove excess water.
- Apply conditioner, if applicable, through the mid-lengths and ends of the extension hairstyle. Avoid applying conditioner to the root area or on the bonds that attach the extensions.
- Stroke the conditioner into the extension hairstyle in downward movements. Leave the conditioner on the hair for the required time then rinse the hair thoroughly using clean running water. Gently squeeze the extension hair to remove excess water.
- After shampooing and conditioning the extension hair, wrap a towel around the hair and pat gently to remove excess water.
- If applicable, apply a pH-balanced rinse into the mid-lengths and ends of the extension hair. Use an applicator or spray bottle recommended by the product company or stylist.
- Once the rinse has been applied, separate the extensions at the root area before drying. This ensures that the bonds do not stick together and that any loose hairs that may be in the root area are not tangled and entwined with a neighbouring extension.
- Use a hairdryer on a warm heat and dry the bonded root area immediately.
- Once the root and bonds are dry brush the extensions gently from the ends towards the root area in a downward direction.
- Hair extensions must be completely dry and placed in a loose plait secured with a covered band on the ends before going to bed at night.
- Always hold extensions at the root area when brushing to avoid unnecessary tension at the roots. Do not apply unnecessary tension to the bonded extension areas by tying ponytails too tight.
- Do not backcomb or backbrush real extension hair as the cuticle layers will interlock and tangling will occur.
- Do not perm or colour real extensions after application because the extension hair has already gone through several chemical processes and any further chemical treatments will result in unpredictable colour or perming results.
- Always remove hair extensions after three months' wear and return to your extension practitioner for this service.

REMEMBER

During the shampooing and conditioning process, do not rub the real extension hair together, as this will cause matting: the cuticle layers will lock together.

ADDITIONAL HOMECARE ADVICE FOR FIBRE EXTENSIONS

- Dry fibre with a warm hairdryer, using a diffuser if required. Hairdryers, airstylers and heated rollers can be used on fibre extension hair.
- When blow-drying fibre extension hair use brushes recommended by a practitioner.
- Fibre extensions cannot be permed or coloured. They are synthetic pre-coloured acrylic fibres, not real human hair; therefore these chemical processes have absolutely no effect on the fibre extension hair.

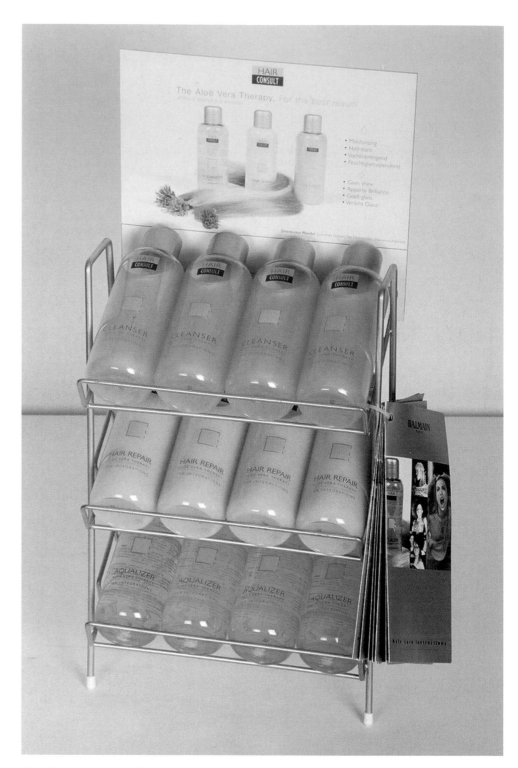

Pierre Balmain, courtesy of Euro Hair Fashion, world licensed manufacturer of Balmain Hair Extensions

As explained in Chapter 3, there are specific aftercare products that are to be in place in a business to recommend and sell to clients.

Some aftercare products are specifically designed to work with either fibre extension hair or real extension hair. The table on the following page shows which products are suitable for the hair product or system chosen to create an extension hairstyle.

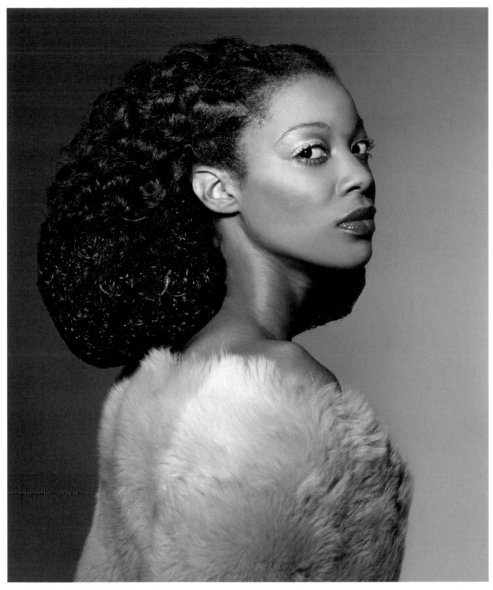

Hair by Kathryn Longmuir at Ishoka, Aberdeen, photography Jim Crone, make-up by Karen Lockyer, clothes styling Kelly Cooper Barr

Products	Notes
A clarifying shampoo	Use this shampoo on every extension system and application
Rinse-out reconstructive conditioner	Use this on real extension hair and fibre extension hair
De-tangling spray	Use to detangle fibre hair
Equalising or PH balanced solutions	Use on real extension hair
Leave-in conditioner	Use on real extension hair
Soft bristle brush	To be used with all extension systems and hairstyles

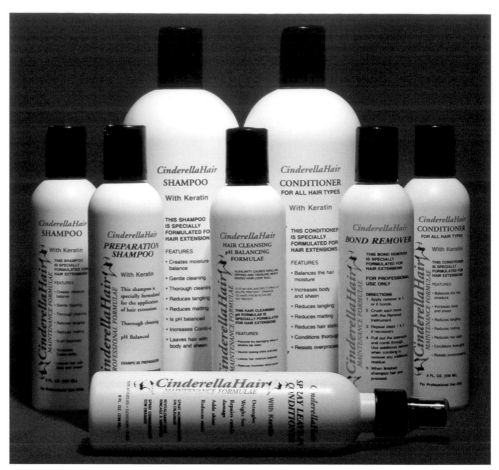

Cinderella

Aftercare advice is as important as the consultation given before extensions are applied. Cover client aftercare procedures during a consultation as this enables the client to make an informed decision to go ahead with this service.

There are many aftercare do's and don'ts to consider when wearing an extension hairstyle:

1 If extensions are shampooed within the 24-hour period of time, bedding-in period, the shampooing and conditioning process will soften the bonds and the extensions will slide out.

2 Do not use brushes with balls on the end of the bristles as these brushes will rip and tear at the extension hair.

3 Brush extension hairstyles thoroughly before shampooing, as this will remove any debris from the extension hairstyle and brush out any loose hairs that may be trapped between the bonds and in between the extension hair.

4 Do not brush extensions when the bonds are wet. When extension bonds are wet they are in their weakest state as most of the extension bonds are porous and will absorb water. Water will make the bonds swell and it is important to dry these swollen bonds very quickly. If water is left in the bonds they can crumble and break and the extensions could slide out.

TOP TIP ✔

Bring the client back into the salon for their first shampoo of their new extension hairstyle. This appointment is designed to teach the client how to shampoo their hair themselves at home, how to use the aftercare products correctly and how to style their new extension hairstyle.

5 Do not apply conditioner onto bonds directly, as conditioners will soften the extension bonds – the polymer resins – causing the extensions to slide out.

6 Real extension hair has been through several chemical processes; the cuticle layer is often damaged or removed. If the extension hair is rubbed together the cuticle layer will lock. This locking acts like velcro and is extremely difficult to separate! Rubbing will result in matting and tangling.

7 Always hold extensions at the roots while brushing to avoid placing unnecessary tension on the root area.

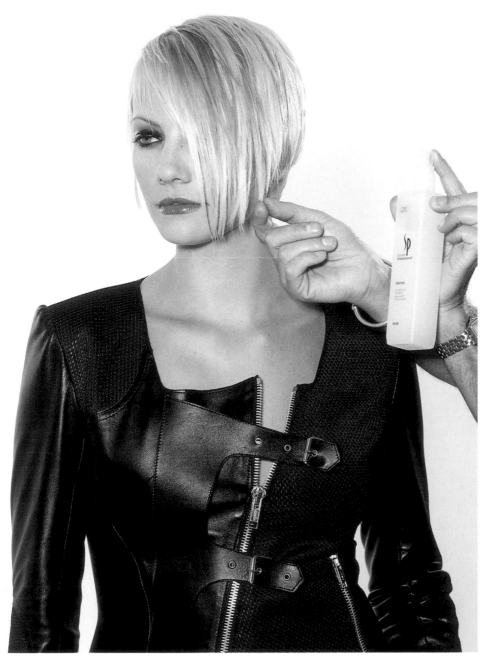

Theresa Bullock

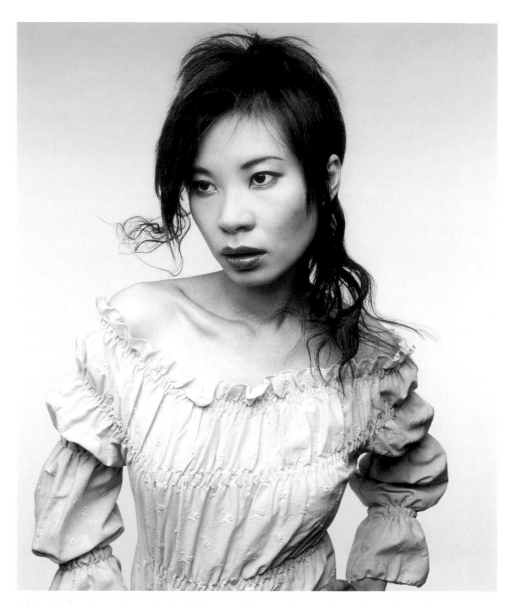

Hair by Rainbow Room International Artistic Team, Glasgow, photography Martin Evening, make-up Janet Francis, clothes styling Angela Barnard

Styling tips for extension hairstyles

- Use styling products recommended by the practitioner.
- Avoid using oil, wax or silicone-based styling products as these chemicals will break the bonds down that hold extensions in place or make natural hair slippery and the extensions will slide out.
- Blow-dry the extension hair thoroughly with a hairdryer using a medium heat. A diffuser can be used.
- A pH-balanced rinse can be used daily before styling and can be applied on wet or dry extension hair.
- Electrical curling tongs, straighteners and hot brushes may be used on real extension hair.
- Always avoid using heated tools on bonded areas, as direct heat will soften the bonds.

- Do not use curling tongs, curling brushes, straighteners or crimpers or any heated electrical hairdressing appliance on fibre extension hair. The heat from these electrical appliances is too excessive for the synthetic fibre hair. It will melt the fibre and damage the surface, which is irreparable.

- Heat will straighten or curl fibre extensions. Once heated and cooled down, the fibre will retain this new straighter or curlier structure until more heat is applied.

- Water will not alter the movement of fibre extensions. Heated rollers will re-curl fibre hair.

- Styling products such as gels and pomades – a wax for example – can be used on dreadlocks or the textured hairstyles to keep the surface smooth so that they do not matt and tangle.

- Remember always remove hair extensions after three months' wear. Return to your stylist for this service.

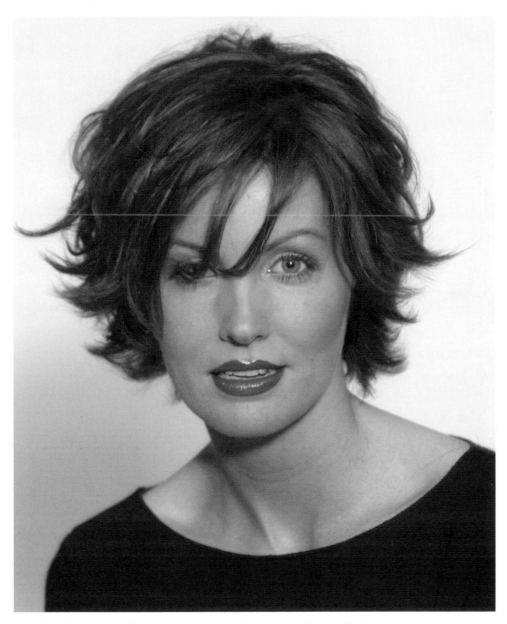

Pierre Balmain, courtesy of Euro Hair Fashion, world licensed manufacturer of Balmain Hair Extensions

Knowledge review

1 What is a client aftercare sheet?

2 List the products to be used when cleansing extension hair.

3 When should an extension hairstyle be shampooed for the first time and why?

4 Why is it important to brush extensions thoroughly before shampooing?

5 What will happen to extensions if they are rubbed together whilst shampooing?

6 Why is it important to separate bonds before shampooing?

7 Why are bonds dried immediately after shampooing and conditioning?

8 Why are extensions tied up at night?

9 What will happen to fibre if it is permed or coloured?

10 What styling products can be used on extension hairstyles?

chapter 10

REMOVING HAIR EXTENSIONS

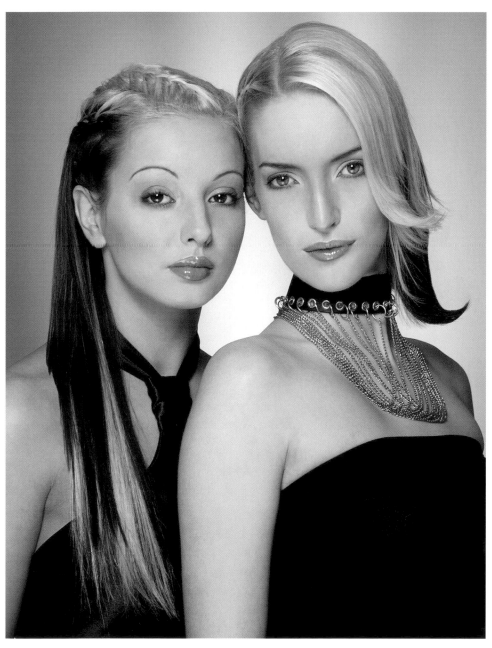

Hair by Aphrodite, Falkirk and Peter and Bernard, Bathgate, photography Jim Crone

INTRODUCTION

All extension systems must be removed at the end of a three-month period of time. The reason for this is every person every day loses 80–100 hairs per day in natural hair fall. Whilst wearing extensions this hair fall cannot come out, and becomes trapped between the scalp and bond of the extension. After three months this natural hair fall will begin to entwine and matt at the root area. This tangling becomes very difficult to remove without causing stress and **breakage** of the natural hair.

> **TOP TIP**
>
> Extensions can be removed and re-applied on the same day. Apply the new extensions above or below the previous extension section – this will help prevent damage to the natural hair.

HEALTH AND SAFETY

Always use the correct extension removal solution with the extension system applied. Always follow the manufacturer's instructions for use of the recommended removal product.

Removing extensions must be conducted professionally and carefully.

The removal procedure is a service which must be scheduled and charged for. Allocate 1–2 hours and prepare a workstation and the environment for this service.

THE TOOLS AND PRODUCTS REQUIRED

HEALTH AND SAFETY

Removal solutions contain strong chemicals. Some solutions can remove nail varnish, nail extensions and cause skin irritation and allergies. It is vital to always wear protective gloves.

- Protective latex gloves or rubber gloves
- A removal tool
- The appropriate extension removal solution
- Cottonwool pads
- A comb and a soft bristle brush.

Each extension system has a different removal procedure. Using the models that are featured in Chapter 8, we explain below the removal procedures for each extension system.

REMOVALS

Kaori removal – a cold-fusion system by Hair Development UK Ltd

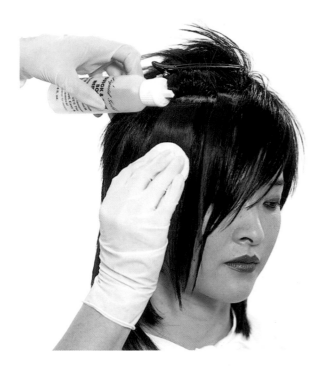

Place a cottonwool pad next to the scalp underneath the weft of extension hair. Apply the removal solution for this system directly onto the weft of extension hair; the cottonwool will catch drips. Using the dampened cottonwool pad, wipe the solution evenly across the weft, leave the solution to penetrate through the weft and onto the natural hair for one minute.

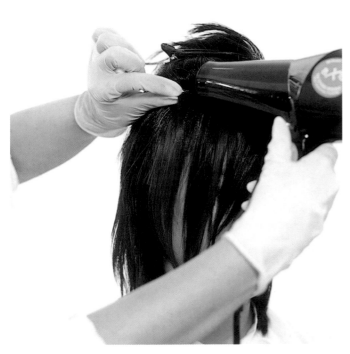

Using a hairdryer heat the weft at the root area for three minutes. Heat activates the removal solution, breaking down the cold-fusion adhesive.

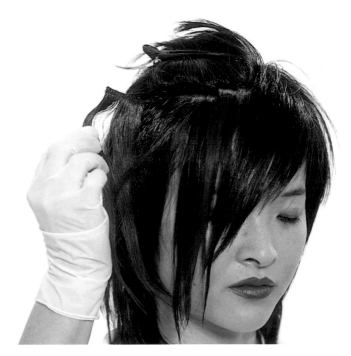

Once the adhesive is softened the weft is ready to peel off. Remove the weft carefully, reapplying removal solution where applicable.

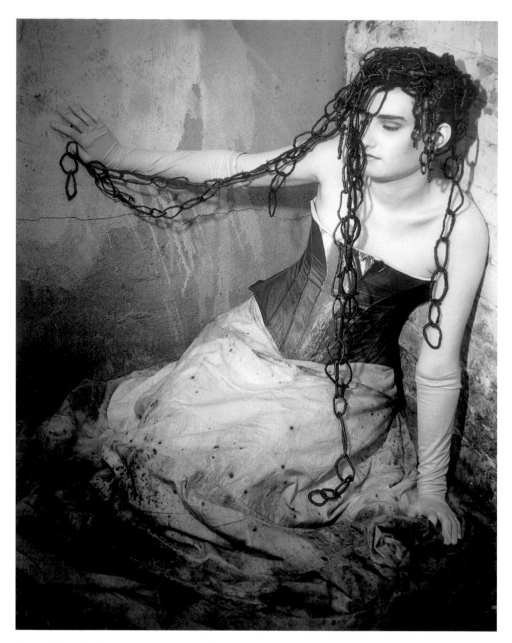

Hair by Jackie Mc Shannon, photography Anders

Removal – hot-bond systems

The hot-bond extension systems all have identical removal procedures. The differences for removal are the recommended removal solutions and removal tools.

Angel removal – for Mane Connection

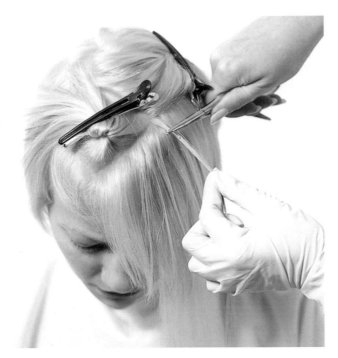

Take a removal tool and crush along the length of the bond.

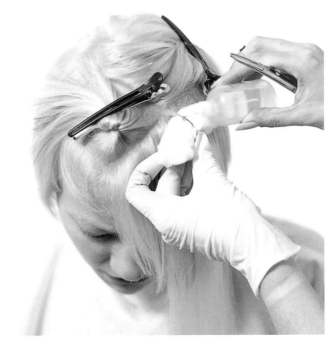

Place a cottonwool pad underneath the bond, to catch any drips of solution. Apply removal solution to the bond fold the cottonwool pad over the bond and hold it for 1–3 minutes; this allows the solution to penetrate the bond.

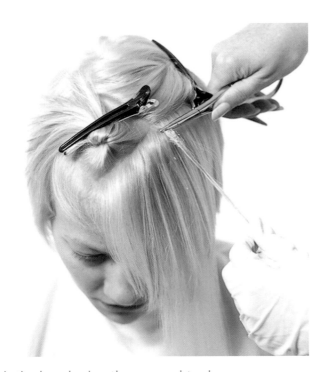

Crush the bond using the removal tool.

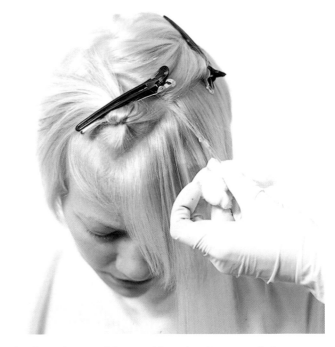

As the bonds crumbles and breaks down pull the extension hair gently away from the natural hair.

Fay removal – for Racoon International

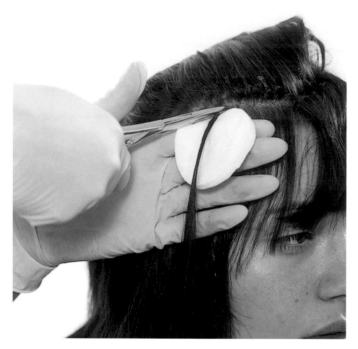

Place a cottonwool pad underneath the extension bond. Apply the removal solution for this resin.

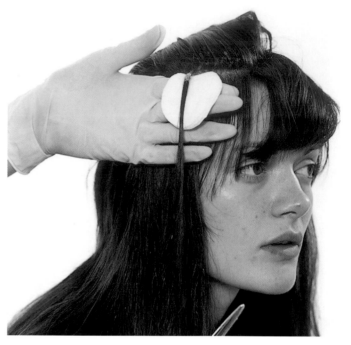

Keeping the pad in place, apply pressure to either side of the bond with a removal tool. The bond is broken in three places: at the top, middle and bottom.

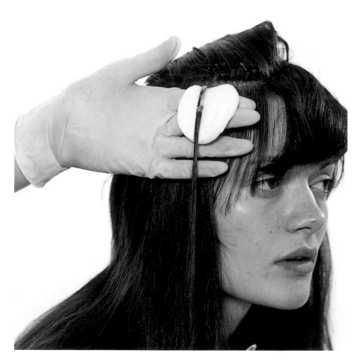

Holding the natural hair at the root, pull the extension strand at the end point for a clean removal.

Laura removal – for Piere Balmain Extensions

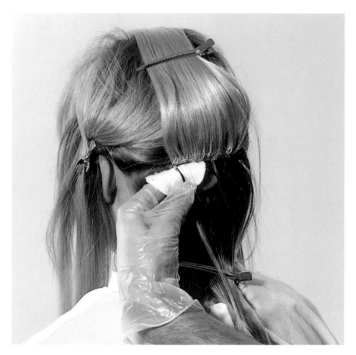

Pin the hair strip out of the way to expose the five strands of natural hair.

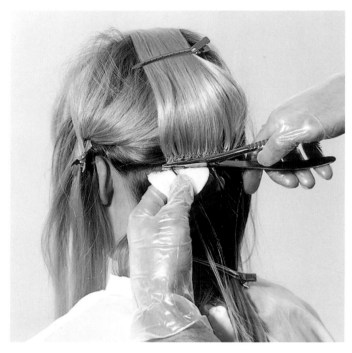

Place a cottonwool pad underneath the first bond and apply removal solution.

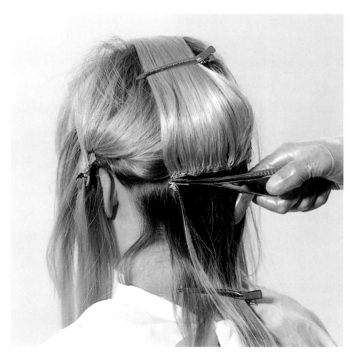

Crush the bond with a removal tool. This is repeated for all five bonds and the hair strip is then pulled away from the natural hair.

Kamilla removal – for Cinderella Hair

This is a pre-bonded extension removal and the procedure does not differ from the three hot-bond extension systems above. Note that the removal tool is of a different design and there is a specific removal solution for the protein moulded bonds used with this company.

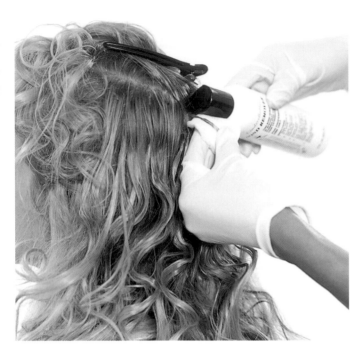

Kamilla removal – step 1

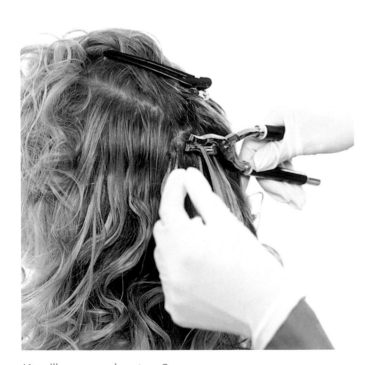

Kamilla removal – step 2

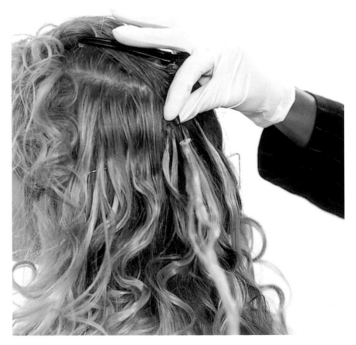

Kamilla removal – step 3

Mia removal – a cold-fusion system using adhesive tapes

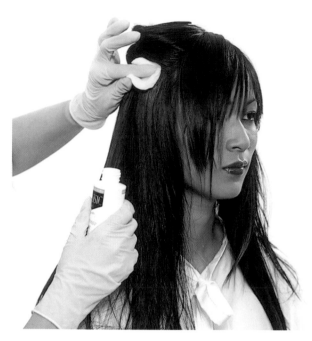

Pour a small amount of the removal solution onto a cottonwool pad. Wipe the top side of the tape near the root area then lift the tape weft and wipe the underside of the weft.

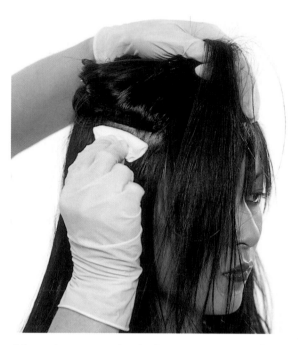

Allow the removal solution to penetrate for 30 seconds to one minute.

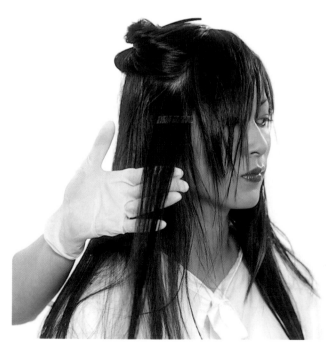

Hold the end of the extension hair contained in the tape and gently pull it away from the hair and scalp. The weft comes away easily from the natural hair in a matter of seconds.

Nina removal – a sewing extension system

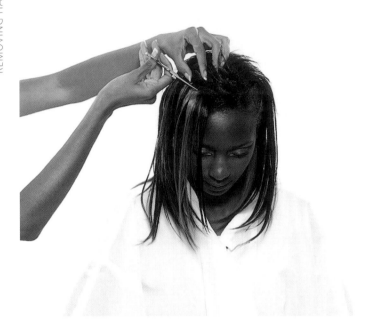

Using old hairdressing scissors carefully cut the stitches that hold the weft in place. The weft will fall from the natural hair.

Jonathon removal – hair alternatives

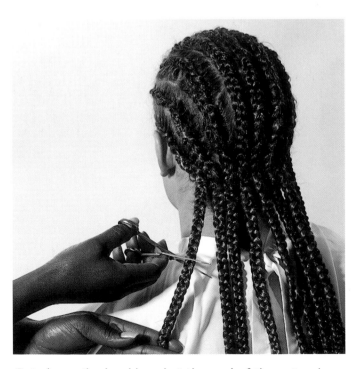

Cut above the hard bond at the end of the extension braid with an old pair of hairdressing scissors.

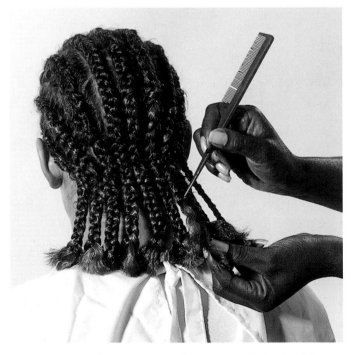

Use the end of a pintail comb to unravel the braid.

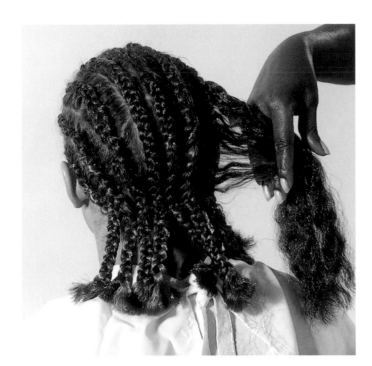

After removing extensions, brush, then comb the natural hair thoroughly to release loose hair and bond debris. Shampoo the natural hair with a clarifying shampoo.

REMOVAL TIPS

- A hair extension hairstyle will prevent natural hair fall. The hair that gets trapped at the root area can cause the natural hair to tangle. To assist you in de-tangling the hair, ask the client to apply conditioner to the bonds the night before removal and to leave it in overnight. The conditioner will help break down the bonds as well as assisting in combing out any tangles.
- If reapplying extensions on the same day as the removal, shampoo the natural hair with a clarifying shampoo prior to reapplication to remove any traces of conditioner. Ensure the client's natural hair is dry and free of any conditioning or styling products before reapplication.

HEALTH AND SAFETY

- Some of the removal solutions are highly flammable. Ensure that nobody smokes in the vicinity and that there are no naked flames near while using the flammable removal solutions.
- While using removal solutions the working area must be well-ventilated.
- Shampoo natural hair thoroughly after using extension removal solutions.
- Do not pour the extension removal solutions on the client's scalp. To prevent the removal solutions coming into contact with the client's scalp use a cottonwool pad to catch any drips.
- All hair extensions must be removed after three months' wear.

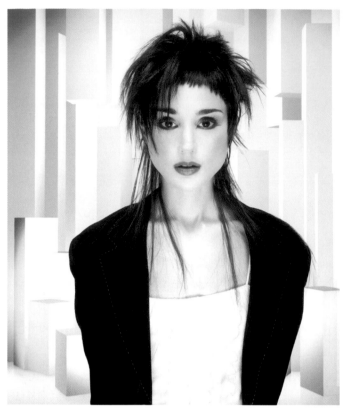

Hair by Stuart Phillips Creative Team, photography Marcello Benfield

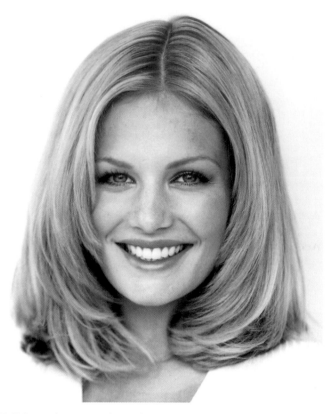

DOME (www.domecosmetics.com)

Knowledge review

1 Why are extensions removed after three months' wear?

2 List the tools and products required for the removal service.

3 Describe the removal procedure of the hot-bond extension system.

4 Why must you work in a well-ventilated area when removing extensions?

5 Why is it imperative to wear protective gloves when removing extensions?

6 What protective clothing should clients wear when removing extensions?

7 Why is the natural hair shampooed after removal?

8 What is used to prevent removal solutions from dropping onto a client's scalp?

9 Can extensions be reapplied after removal?

10 What are the two removal tips itemised in this chapter?

glossary of terms

Accident book a notebook where any salon accidents are recorded.

Acetone a colourless volatile liquid ketone used as a solvent. Some extension removal solutions contain acetone; therefore great care must be taken when using them. The COSHH outlines the steps that need to be taken when handling hazardous substances.

Acrylic a man-made synthetic fibre or fabric.

African-Caribbean hair the very curly hair typical of African-Caribbean people.

Aftercare products the product clients require to look after their extension hairstyle. These products are specific to the particular extension system and product that have been used to create the hairstyle.

Aftercare requirements these include the products the client needs to use on their extension hairstyle, styling instructions and maintenance appointments (including the removal appointment).

Airstyler a low-powered hairdryer and brush combined, ideal for styling extension hairstyles.

Alcohol a pure spirit.

Allergies clients may have allergic reactions to some of the products used in the hair extension service. This is why it is vital to do strand and sensitivity tests before proceeding with the extension hairstyle.

Alopecia baldness.

Anaphylactic shock when a person is extremely allergic to a substance they can suffer an anaphylactic shock, which can be fatal. Again, strand and sensitivity tests are crucial to test for allergic reactions.

Applicator (hot extension applicator) a tool used with hot-bond systems. It heats pre-bonded extension strands, melting the polymer resin to secure the extension and natural hair at the root area.

Asian hair hair that comes from the Indian continent or nationals of these countries.

Barrier conditioner/barrier cream waterproof cream to protect the skin or scalp when using chemicals.

Base/first colour the colour nearest to the client's natural hair colour

Baseline The perimeter line of a hairstyle. Fibre extension hair should always be chipped into with old hairdressing scissors, rather than cut in a straight line, to create a natural-looking baseline.

Bedding-in period the hair extension hairstyle should be shampooed no earlier than 24 hours after application to allow the bonds to set and harden. This is referred to as the bedding-in period.

Block blending mixing extension hair together with several colours and ensuring that the colours are separated into colour streaks or blocks of colours

Block colouring colouring areas of hair in a way that is intended to enhance the cut style. This technique creates a block colour strip or streaky colour effect.

Bond/hard bond the hardened polymer resin adhesive that attaches extension hair to natural hair.

Bonded root area the area where extensions are attached to natural hair.

Bonding/fusion solutions/bonding adhesive/ bonding tapes are all used with cold-fusion systems.

Braid a technique that entwines several pieces of hair together to create a decorative strand

Braiding extension system *see* Plaiting/braiding extension system.

Breakage when a client's natural hair has been broken off.

Brickwork individual strands of extension hair should be applied in a brickwork fashion so that each row of extensions sits directly above the one before, leaving the extension strand above to fall between two strands below.

Bulk blending/mega-mixing the method of brushing different colour strands of fibre together to match the client's natural hair colour so that the first, second and third colours are all blended together with no stripes visible.

Bulk hair loose real extension hair with a band tied around the root area.

Caucasian hair the wavy or straight hair typical of a European.

Caustic soda (sodium hydroxide) is used to cleanse real extension hair in order to remove any infestations before it reaches the salon; it is a corrosive product.

Clarifying shampoo a deep-cleansing shampoo that removes residues, oils and waxes. It should be used on the natural hair prior to applying extensions and throughout the duration of the extension hairstyle.

Client aftercare procedures these are the instructions that the client is given to enable them to care for their new extension hairstyle.

Client consultation sheet is a sheet that details the planning of the extension hairstyle, from the desired hairstyle to maintenance appointments. The practitioner and the client should each have a copy of this sheet and both need to sign it at the end of the consultation.

Closely scattered placement putting one extension next to another in a row, leaving a $\frac{1}{4}-\frac{1}{2}$ cm gap of loose natural hair between each extension. This placement gives root lift, volume and thickness.

Cold adhesives/cold solutions products used with cold-fusion systems.

Cold fusing using cold-fusion products to attach extension hair to natural hair.

Cold-fusion extension systems extension systems whereby extension hair is attached to natural hair using products, such as spirit/latex/rubber-based gums or toupee tapes.

Cold solutions *see* cold adhesives.

Colour formula is a guideline used when mixing and blending extension hair to match the client's natural hair colour. It is a similar principle to mixing tints for adding mixed tones.

Colour rings/colour shade charts holds swatches of extension hair colours. This can be placed next to the client's natural hair when selecting the extension hair colour/s.

Colours (fibre) natural colours, tonal colours, fantasy colours, neon colours, pre-blended colours.

Colours (real) pure virgin natural colours – real extension hair that has not been bleached or tinted, tinted natural colours, tinted tonal colours, two-tone colours.

Consultation a process of communication in which the client expresses their wishes and the hairdresser gives advice.

Contra-indication a reason why a proposed course of action or treatment should not be pursued because it may be inadvisable or harmful.

Cornrows/cornbraids/scalp plaits fine plaits running continuously across the scalp. Fibre can be braided into them as an extension hairstyle. They also contain and condense the natural hair so that weaves or wefts may be sewn into them.

COSHH Control of Substances Hazardous to Health Act 1999.

Cross-infection the passing of an infection from one individual to another.

Curly the name for real hair that has such a strong S-shaped bend throughout the length that it folds over and curls.

Curved needle and thread are used to sew wefts onto natural hair.

Cuticle correct *see* Root point perfect.

Cuticle layers the protective layer covering hair. The chemical treatments that real extension hair has undergone can often damage the natural cuticle layer. A pH-balanced/equalising solution should be used on real extension hair to close the cuticle layers. Shampooing in a shower is also important to prevent these damaged cuticle layers from locking together, which can result in matting and tangling.

Deep wave a brand name for real hair that has a strong S-shaped bend throughout the length.

Defect in the equipment salon owners and managers are responsible for the maintenance of their equipment. A record card should be kept listing the dates of purchase, repair and replacement of all equipment.

Dermatitis inflammation of the skin.

De-tangling spray reduces tangling and static electricity on fibre extension hair. It should be used daily.

Diamond crystal crystal gems cut in the shape of a diamond stone.

Directionally place/directional work the practitioner should place extensions in the direction of the natural hair, so that it falls naturally and blends with the natural hair.

Dispenser (hot-bond extension dispenser) this hot-bond tool works by depositing a hot polymer resin adhesive at the root end of the extension hair, attaching both resin and extension hair onto the natural hair.

Dreadlocks long thin texture of hair that is created by matting or tangling natural or fibre hair together.

Eczema an inflammation of the skin, characterised by redness and irritation.

Electricity at Work Regulations 1989 it is important to pay close attention to these regulations when working in a salon. All electrical equipment should be checked regularly by a qualified electrician.

Enzyme treatment a treatment on real extension hair, promoted by product companies, enabling the real extension hair to be tinted.

Equalising a normalising solution that restores real hair back to its normal state.

European hair hair that comes from European countries or nationals of that region.

Extension placement how the practitioner places the extensions. There are five types of placement: solid/continuous row, closely scattered, scattered, visual and weft.

Extension practitioner stylist qualified to apply hair extensions.

Extension size you can make several different extension sizes depending on the system that you are working with and the hairstyle that you want to create. For all extension sizes, the ratio of extension hair to natural hair is always the same: 50 per cent extension hair to 50 per cent natural hair.

Fantasy colours unnatural or pure colours, e.g. royal blue, banana yellow, poppy red.

Fibre braids three- or four-stem braids made of fibre extension hair.

Finger razor a finger tool with a razor at the end for tapering the ends of the hair.

First aid kit should include all of the basic first aid requirements for a salon. All staff must know where it is kept.

Flammable easily set on fire.

Flat stable work surface is vital when working with hot-bond extension systems. Heated tools need to be kept on a flat stable surface at all times to avoid unnecessary accidents. It is not advisable to place hot tools on hairdressing trolleys, as they can be unstable.

Flat tapering technique a cutting technique using a razor, leaving the natural hair with a very fine soft perimeter edge.

Four-stem braid/four-stem locking braid/ backcombed four-stem braid two practitioners are required to create this braid: a stylist and an assistant. Backcombed fibre is braided into the natural hair to create a radical alternative look.

Further education colleges training for the hair extension service can be obtained at some further education colleges.

Gaslift chair/hydraulic chair chairs suitable for the hair extension service. As this service can take many hours, it important that the client sits in a chair that can be moved up and down so that the practitioner can avoid repetitive strain injury.

Hair additions this extension hairstyle consists of extension strands attached to a client's natural hairstyle to create highlights, lowlights and flashes of colour, decorations and adornments.

Hair alternatives this extension hairstyle is created using textured fibre or real extension hair made into braids or dreadlocks. Alternatives completely cover natural hairstyles and are seen as radical changes to a client's image.

Hair analysis examination of the hair.

Hair colour the extension hair should be matched to the client's natural hair prior to ordering as, in general, extension hair should not be coloured. Chemical treatments have no affect on fibre hair and real extension hair has already undergone chemical treatments.

Hair enhancements this extension hairstyle is created using extension hair that matches the client's natural hair colour to thicken the natural hair and improve the look of the natural hairstyle.

Hair extension real or synthetic fibre added to existing hair.

Hair extension hairstyle a hair extensions hairstyle is one where the client's existing hair is lengthened using real or fibre extension hair.

Hair extension service a service provided by a salon whereby extension hair (either real or fibre) is applied into natural hair to create a variety of different extension hairstyles.

Hair extension systems are the different systems used by the extension practitioner to apply extension hair onto natural hair. They include hot-bond and cold-fusion systems, as well as braiding and plaiting and sewing systems.

Hair fall we lose 80–100 hairs every day. This is called natural hair fall.

Hair length and density the length above or below the shoulders, the amount of hair on the head and the thickness of the individual hairs. For an extension hairstyle, the client's hair must never be extended by more than twice their natural hair length.

Hair strip a small pre-prepared weft of hair.

Hair texture the feel of the hair: fine, medium or coarse. For a natural-looking extension hairstyle, the texture of the extension hair must always match the texture of the client's natural hair.

Hard bond *see* bond.

HASAWA Health and Safety at Work Act 1974.

Health and safety legislation it is essential to follow all health and safety legislation. This is absolutely vital when dealing with technical hairdressing services, like the hair extension service, where strong chemicals and heated tools are used.

Health and safety policy the manager of the salon is required by law to draw up a health and safety policy for their salon. Each employee must be given a copy of this policy and ensure that they understand it fully.

Heat clamp this tool is used with hot-bond systems to heat fibre extension hair. It melts the fibre surrounding the natural hair together, forming a hard bond at the root area.

Heat sealing using a heat clamp to seal the ends of fibre or to seal a pre-bonded extension strand.

Hot-bond/hot melt extension systems use a variety of heated tools to attach extension hair onto natural hair, such as applicators, dispensers and clamps.

Insurance cover all salons must obtain full insurance cover before introducing the hair extension service.

Interlock lock together.

Isosceles triangle a triangle shape with two equal sides.

Jumbo fibre a type of fibre extension hair commonly used in braiding, particularly for clients with African-Caribbean hair textures.

Keratin the principle protein of hair, nails and skin.

Knot/rosebud smooth dreadlocks are twisted to form these knots that look like rosebuds. They are ideal for strong avant-garde looks, as well as bridal hairstyles.

Latex or rubber gloves must be worn when handling strong chemicals, such as those found in removal solutions.

Leave-in conditioner is designed to moisturise and condition natural hair and real extension hair. It should not be applied onto the adhesives or the bonded root area.

Legal requirements as with any business, there are certain legal requirements when offering hairdressing services.

Liable for negligence means that the practitioner must take full responsibility for failing to take proper care.

Liquid gold type of spirit gum used with cold-fusion systems. It can be painted on to the thread of a weft to attach it to the natural hair.

Maintenance appointments tidy-up, fill-in, removal: these maintenance appointments are essential when wearing a hair extension hairstyle and should be booked in advance.

Major tone/second colour is the second nearest colour to the client's natural hair colour.

Matting of extension hair can occur with both real and fibre extension hair, usually this is because the correct aftercare procedures are being ignored.

Mclau a finger tool used for sectioning hair, allowing the practitioner to take straight clean sections of hair.

Mega-mixing *see* bulk blending.

Microbonding when working on a triangular section, extension strands can be applied to the top and bottom of the longest point of the isosceles triangle to build up weight in the hairstyle.

Minor tone/third colour this colour may only appear as tiny strands of colour in a client's natural hair, such as a percentage of white hair.

Mixing and blending is the process of mixing and blending extension hair to match the client's natural hair colour. For fibre, the different colour strands are simply brushed together. A mixing mat is used for real extension hair.

Mixing mat a 12 cm × 12 cm flat mat with small metal teeth used to blend real extension hair.

Negligence carelessness or lack of proper care and attention.

Neon colours colours that glow under ultra violet lights.

Non-porous a non-porous material will not allow water or air to penetrate. Man-made materials, such as synthetic fibre, are non-porous.

Non-refundable deposits assure the client that there will be a stylist available to perform the extension hairstyle and also assure the stylist that lost revenue will be recovered if the client does not turn up. The client must be given a receipt for this deposit.

Occipital bone bone forming the back of the head.

Oil a thick liquid substance that is sticky and lubricates.

Oriental hair hair that comes from the Orient, for example China, or nationals of that region.

pH-balanced pH is a table used to gage the acidity or alkalinity of a solution. This solution restores the real hair to the same acidity as natural hair.

pH-balanced/equalising solution is designed to close the cuticle layers of real extension hair to reduce matting and tangling.

pH scale measure of acidity or alkalinity.

Plaiting/braiding extension systems are extension systems whereby fibre is plaited or braided into the natural hair using cornbraids or scalp plaits.

Polymer a compound of a complex molecule formed by the combination of identical molecules.

Polymer resin adhesive sticks are used with hot-bond dispensers. Different adhesive sticks are used with different dispensers. Always use adhesive sticks that have been recommended by the company that supplied the dispenser.

Porosity the ability to hold moisture.

Porous having minute holes/spaces through which liquid or air may pass.

Practical training it is essential to have practical training as well as learning the underpinning knowledge before introducing the hair extension service to your business.

Pre-bonded strand a strand of extension hair that has a polymer resin already attached to the root end.

Private extension training companies independent tuition centres that are not attached to product companies.

Psoriasis a condition that produces inflammation, irritation and scaling of the skin.

Public and Employers Liability insurance cover for businesses who service the general public and employ staff.

Real human extension hair/real hair/natural extension hair is real human Asian, Oriental or European hair prepared for extension hairstyles. It can be bought as individual strands, on a weft or as bulk hair. It is more expensive than fibre extension hair and, because it is scarce, European hair is the most expensive real extension hair on the market.

Reconstructive conditioner a conditioner that works inside the structure of the hair shaft to strengthen it. It should be used to care for real extension hair.

Rectangular sections are available in two sizes: $1/2$ cm wide × 1 cm deep or 1 cm wide × 2 cm deep. They are suitable for curly, African-Caribbean hair or very thick hair. The rectangular section condenses the root area, reducing bulk to prevent a distorted or misshapen hairstyle.

Re-growth application colouring the natural hair that has grown since the last treatment with colour or bleach.

Removal all extensions must be removed after three months. The removal appointment and all other maintenance appointments should be booked ahead of time. Clients should not attempt to remove extensions at home.

Removal solutions these solutions are applied to the extension bonds to break them down.

Removal tool like a pair of pliers and is used to crush the bonds attaching the extension hair once the solution has fully penetrated the bond.

Repetitive strain injury condition in which the prolonged performance of repetitive actions causes pain or impairment of functions in the tendons and muscles involved. Extension practitioners need to be aware of this as some extension applications take many hours to perform. Wearing appropriate clothing, shoes and using adjustable chairs will help to prevent this condition.

Resin an adhesive, a secretion of trees or plants. Hot-bond extension dispensers deposit polymer resins onto the end of extension hair. The polymer resin is inserted into the tool. Polymer resins are produced on the end of extension hair when working with pre-bonded extensions.

Ringlet curl the name for real hair that has such a strong S-shaped bend throughout the length that it folds over and creates a curl stretching down the length of long hair. Ringlets are flat curls, created by winding the hair flat around a rod, curler or rag.

Roll the adhesive the adhesive bond has to be rolled to seal it. When dealing with hot adhesives it is essential to use a silicone pad to protect your fingers.

Root the base of the hair.

Root point perfect/cuticle correct extensions must always be applied root point perfect, with the root of the extension strand or weft placed at the root area of the natural hair. Placing extensions in upside down can cause severe tangling and matting that can be almost impossible to remove.

Scalp protectors/scalp shields are small discs with a hole in the centre designed to draw out strands of natural hair. They protect the scalp from all heated tools and hot polymer resins.

Scalp sensitivity pain or tenderness in the scalp.

Scalp tension the amount of pulling at the scalp.

Scattered placement where the practitioner puts one extension next to another in a row, leaving a $1/2$–1 cm gap of loose natural hair in between. It can be used to create highlights or lowlights.

Sebum oily secretion of a sebaceous gland, causing greasy hair.

Section $1/2$ cm square this small extension size is used with hot-bond systems and enables the practitioner to create an extension hairstyle where the attachments are undetectable.

Section 1 cm square used for braiding extension hair into natural hair. This larger extension size is suitable for braiding as a wider circumference of hair is required for this technique.

Section 2 cm square this extension size is used when applying hair alternatives such as dreadlocks, because a greater quantity of natural hair is required to hold the textured extension without putting any strain on the natural hair.

Sensitivity tests are essential to ensure that the client is not allergic to any of the products used in the extension system that you are applying.

Separate the bonds clients must separate extension bonds before shampooing to prevent hair entwining at the root area as this can cause the bonds to lock together and tangling will occur.

Sewing extension system is where wefts are applied onto cornbraids or twists using a curved needle and silk thread.

Sharps box the designated box in a salon into which all used razors are deposited for disposal.

Shedding hair that falls off or falls out.

Silicone pads are small pieces of silicone that the practitioner uses to protect their fingers when rolling the hot bond.

Silky straight a brand name for straight real hair.

Skin sensitivity tests tests that check whether a client is allergic to the products that are used to attach extensions.

Smooth dreadlocks a dreadlock that has a smooth surface.

Soft bristle brush used to brush through the client's natural and extension hair. It should be used daily to get rid of loose hair, therefore reducing tangling and matting.

Soft wave a brand name for real hair that has a gentle S-shaped bend throughout the length.

Solid/continuous row of extensions where extensions are placed next to each other, giving a blanket or sheet of hair. This placement provides bulk and thickness.

Spiral tapering is a method of layering the hair without removing any of the length. The hair is taken in small sections and sliced into at the three points of the twist. This is ideal for removing blunt lines before applying extensions.

Spiral wave the name for real hair that has such a strong S-shaped bend throughout the length that it folds over and creates a curl stretching down the length of long hair.

Spirit/latex/rubber-based gums are all types of cold-fusion solutions used to attach extension hair.

Spirit gum/anti-slipping agent prevents fibre from slipping out of Caucasian, Asian and Oriental hair types.

Sticks wrapping fibre around a four-stem locking braid creates smooth dreadlocks, sometimes called sticks.

Strand test a strand test must be performed on all clients before attempting to apply extensions. This is to check that the client's natural hair is strong enough and that the extensions will not slip out.

Strands of extension hair/individual extension strands these are usually applied using hot-bond systems and give a very natural, free-flowing look.

Strips see weaves.

Structures (fibre) straight hair, soft wave, deep wave, curly, spiral, ringlets, dreadlocks, crimped, crinkly, braided, zigzag, tight Afro curl, relaxed African-Caribbean texture, Yaki hair. These are the various structures available for fibre extension hair.

Structures (real) silky straight, soft wave, deep wave, curly, spiral curl, ringlet. These are the various structures available for real extension hair.

Synthetic fibre extension hair/fibre is a man-made fibre specifically designed to create wigs, hairpieces and hair extensions. It can be bought as individual extension strands, on a weft or as bulk hair. It is non-porous acrylic so chemical treatments will have no effect on it.

Tail comb a comb with an extension that is useful for sectioning and guiding hair.

Tapered thinner towards the hair points.

Tapering cutting a hair section to a tapered point (i.e. a point like that of a sharpened pencil).

Tapes see toupee tapes.

Tensile strength the strength of the hair when it is under strain or stretched.

Tension the stress or stretch experienced by hair.

Tension spots/discomfort can occur, particularly on Caucasian hair types, if appropriate care has not been taken with tensioning.

Texture the feel or appearance of the hair – rough, smooth, coarse or fine.

Textured shaped to take account of the fineness or coarseness of hair, giving lift and fullness.

Textured fibre braid/dreadlock these are usually used in alternative extension hairstyles and can either be bought pre-prepared or created in the salon using fibre extension hair. The fibre can be backcombed to create particular textures.

Thinning reducing the bulk of hair without reducing its length.

Thread/rose wire/beads are used to seal the end of a braid to prevent unravelling. Polymer resins or cold-fusion spirit gums can also be used.

Three-stem braid is a braid created by braiding fibre into the client's natural hair.

Tinted fantasy colours chemical colour added to create fantasy hair colour.

Tinted natural colours chemical colours added to look like natural hair colour.

Tinted tonal colours chemical colour added to give a tone of hair colour.

Toupee tapes adhesive tapes used with some cold-fusion systems to attach wefts of extension hair.

Traction stress or pull applied to the hair.

Traction alopecia an area of baldness resulting from the stress or pull applied to hair.

Triangular sections come in two sizes: $\frac{1}{2}$ cm or 1 cm wide. Triangular sections are preferred by some of the product companies, as the section shape is more suitable for their application technique.

Twists sometimes used instead of cornbraids for a quicker extension application. This works well on African-Caribbean hair. The hair is sectioned in rows and simply twisted and fixed with a hold-in spray. Wefts can then be sewn onto the twists.

Two-tone colours two colours are seen on one strand of hair; one colour at the root area and one colour at the end of the hair.

Underpinning knowledge the theoretical knowledge a student needs along with practical training for the hair extension service.

Virgin hair hair that has never been treated by any chemical process.

Virgin natural colours having no chemicals added to alter the colour, or natural colour.

Visual placement is where the practitioner examines the completed hairstyle and places small extensions where gaps appear or where blending is required.

Water-soluble a substance that will break down and rinse away in water.

Weaves/wefts/hair strips/wefted hair strips of real or fibre extension hair, not unlike a sheet or curtain of hair. They can be sewn into the natural hair or applied using hot-bond or cold-fusion systems.

Wefts see weaves.

Weft placement is relevant when applying weaves or wefts. A weft placement either overrides the existing hairstyle or is incorporated into the interior of the hairstyle. It can only ever achieve solid placement.

Well ventilated because some of the application and removal solutions for the hair extension service contain very strong chemicals, it is very important that the salon is well ventilated as the smell of chemicals can make you feel nauseous.

index